Published by eddyjoemd, LLC.

This book is available in print and digital format on Amazon.com.

ISBN: 979-8-8592-5820-8

Printed in the United States by Amazon.com

THE VASOPRESSOR & INOTROPE HANDBOOK

A PRACTICAL GUIDE FOR HEALTHCARE PROFESSIONALS

BY EDDY J. GUTIERREZ, MD

@EDDYJOEMD

DISCLAIMER

The information in this book—*The Vasopressor & Inotrope Handbook: A Practical Guide for Healthcare Professionals*—is intended for informational purposes only. It is not a substitute for professional medical advice, diagnosis, or treatment. The content provided in this book is meant to be a general guide and educational resource for medical professionals.

The information presented in this book is based on the author's research and experience up to the publication date. Medical knowledge constantly evolves, and new information may alter the recommendations or understanding of vasopressors and inotropes. Therefore, readers are strongly encouraged to refer to up-to-date medical literature and guidelines to make informed decisions regarding patient care.

The author and the publisher do not make any warranties, express or implied, regarding the accuracy, completeness, or suitability of the information contained in this book. They shall not be held responsible for any errors, omissions, or actions taken based on the information provided in this book.

Readers are advised to use their clinical judgment and seek guidance from appropriate medical experts when making patient care decisions, including using vasopressors and inotropes. This book does not constitute medical advice, and its content should not be considered a replacement for individualized medical assessment and treatment.

The author and publisher of this book disclaim any liability or responsibility for any adverse outcomes or consequences resulting from the use of information contained in this book. The ultimate responsibility for patient care lies with the healthcare provider, who should always exercise due diligence and follow established medical protocols and best practices.

By reading this book, you acknowledge that you have read, understood, and agreed to this disclaimer. If you do not agree with these terms, you should not use this book.

To my late father, whose courage, strength, and unwavering positivity continue to guide me. To my mother, who is the embodiment of resilience, sacrifice, and unwavering love. To my wife, who is my life companion, best friend, my constant support, and the pillar of our family. To my daughters, who inspire and motivate me every day with their love, curiosity, and joy. This book is a tribute to the love and lessons you have all gifted me.

TABLE OF CONTENTS

INTRODUCTION

My Critical Care Origin Story
In July 2012, I started my Internal Medicine residency. Day one found me in the ICU, a setting entirely new to me. My foreign medical school education did not cover critical care. My first encounter with a ventilated patient in the ICU was a jolt of reality. His sudden responsiveness shattered my misconception that ventilated patients were always deeply sedated. The medications, the alarms, the physiology, the ventilator settings—I had much to learn.

Dr. James Ramage, one of the ICU attending physicians, appropriately expressed frustration at my initial presentations. I could sense the vastness of what I needed to learn, coupled with the delicate balance these patients' lives hung on. I remember feeling overwhelmed yet driven to overcome my limitations.

Mentorship played a pivotal role in my journey. Drs. Ramage, Carl Kemp, Stephen Morris, Igor Aksenov, Dominic Roma, and others inspired me to pursue Critical Care Medicine. Conversations with Drs. Kemp and Morris particularly resonated with me, as they saw potential in me I had not yet recognized. Dr. Michael Ruiz was my first advocate, pivotal in my residency acceptance and growth as an internist. Dr. Drew McGregor's invitation to join his critical care fellowship program was a milestone in my career. These mentors, along with family, friends, colleagues, and many others, shaped me into the physician I am today.

My father's influence remains the strongest. His resilience, escaping from Cuba and immigrating to the U.S. instilled in me the value of opportunity and hard work. He always envisioned me as a physician, even when I doubted myself and chose different career paths. His unfortunate diagnosis fueled my desire to make a difference in healthcare. His unwavering belief in me remains a guiding force even after his too-early passing.

Gratitude: A Hat Tip to the Authors
In creating this book, I am acutely aware that I stand on the shoulders of giants. The fundamental essence of this text is built upon the groundbreaking work of countless scientists and researchers whose discoveries have saved millions of lives. Their tireless efforts, encompassing thousands of clinical trials, have advanced our patient management.

This book is my endeavor to synthesize this wealth of data, transforming it into a comprehensive guide on vasopressors and inotropes. I aim to equip you with the knowledge to become proficient in this field without sifting through hundreds of medical journal articles.

I extend my deepest gratitude to everyone whose work is cited here. Your contribution to the families of patients who participated in these clinical trials is invaluable. I offer my heartfelt thanks to the unsung heroes on the research teams, often working tirelessly behind the scenes without public acknowledgment. Thank you to the bedside nurses and pharmacists who meticulously prepare and administer these critical medications. Your role is vital in the seamless execution of these studies and our daily management of patients.

Lastly, if I missed mentioning anyone who participated in this journey, please know your contribution is appreciated. There is an entire world of effort in research that often goes unseen, extending far beyond the names listed below the paper's title.

Acknowledgments

This book is a tribute to the many individuals who have contributed to my growth. Each has left a significant mark on my journey, from mentors and colleagues to family and friends. Special thanks to my wife, Avery, and peers who reviewed and provided invaluable insights, including Casey Bryant, Brian Gardner, Josh Jackson, Haney Mallemat, Tim Mikulas, David Mysona, Mayank Patel, Cody Perrigo, Jordan Reppond, Vishal Singh, Caroline Welch, Patrick Wieruszewski, and Amanda Yassin.

Disclaimer, Approach, and Humility

This book synthesizes extensive reading, lectures, and over a decade of clinical experience. It represents my interpretations of many articles and is not a peer-reviewed textbook. Mistakes will be made in interpreting this evidence. It reflects my ongoing journey in medicine, where learning never ceases.

The format of this book is designed to engage and provoke thought. The question-and-answer style, born from my teaching experiences, aims to foster a deeper understanding of vasopressors and inotropes. This is not a dosing guide but an exploration of key concepts and real-world applications. Some concepts will be repeated in different chapters. This is for those who use this as a reference.

Throughout this book, you will encounter many questions that do not have straightforward, black-and-white answers. This reflects medicine's complex and ever-evolving nature, where absolute certainties are rare and discoveries continually reshape our understanding. Despite these complexities and the vast expanse of the unknown, we strive to make the best decisions based on the data and knowledge currently available to us.

Limitations

Medicine is a field with seemingly endless depths to explore. However, this book aims to avoid diving into these profound depths. Instead, it balances depth and readability, providing enough detail to be informative without overwhelming you, the reader. I intend to maintain your engagement, using my attention span as a barometer for delving into complexity. While I endeavor to provide valuable content, there may be moments where the depth is either lacking or excessive. For example, delving into the minutiae of p-values, confidence intervals, and statistical nuances of every study would undoubtedly enrich the content but at the risk of impeding readability. The target audience is wide.

Randomized controlled trials (RCTs) are fundamental in advancing our understanding of patient management, and various methodologies exist to conduct them, each suited to different research needs. These methodologies range from parallel-group RCTs to placebo-controlled, crossover, cluster, adaptive, and factorial RCTs, among others. Some RCTs are further categorized as multi-center, open-label, etc., offering unique insights into the study's design and execution. I generally refer to these variations in this book as 'RCTs' unless a specific type is particularly relevant to the discussion. For those interested in how a particular RCT was conducted, I encourage you to delve into the original articles. The citations are streamlined to facilitate easy access to these sources, allowing you to explore the intricate details at your convenience.

Chasing Citations
Citations are essential for verifying information and diving deeper into topics. I frequently say, *"Read these articles for yourself, and do not trust me."* To facilitate this, each chapter includes a URL and QR codes leading to my website, where you can find links to articles and additional resources. Many are open-access.

I have selected the National Library of Medicine (NLM) citation format for this book primarily because it includes each article's PubMed ID (PMID). The PMID, typically an 8-digit number, is a direct gateway to the abstract on PubMed when entered into a search engine. This approach simplifies the process of locating source materials for further reading. A few articles cited in this book were sourced from platforms other than PubMed and, as such, do not possess a PMID. Some citations may deviate from standard formats and appear somewhat unconventional. I am open to feedback regarding these citation formats and am willing to make necessary updates for clarity and consistency.

Errata
"If you don't make mistakes, you're not working on hard enough problems. And that's a big mistake" - Frank Wilczek. I will likely make some mistakes in this book. Your corrections and feedback are welcome. Any errors identified will be corrected in future editions and listed at eddyjoemd.com/errata/.

Thank you.

Your support along this journey means everything. I have received so many encouraging messages from you all over the years of support and motivation to keep on pushing forward. I hope not to disappoint. This book aims to deliver value that justifies your investment. It is a culmination of collective efforts, and I hope it serves as a valuable resource in your medical journey. I am ever grateful.

01: THE BASICS

Keeping it simple and still accurate-ish.
To demystify hemodynamics, I turn to a simple yet powerful equation: MAP = (CO x SVR) + CVP.[1] This equation invariably comes to my mind with every hemodynamically unstable patient I encounter. I recommend memorizing it if you have not already done so.

Let's decode these acronyms: MAP is mean arterial pressure, CO is cardiac output, SVR is systemic vascular resistance, and CVP is central venous pressure. If this still seems complex, let's simplify it further. Since CVP often holds a negligible value, sometimes even zero,[10] we frequently reduce the equation to MAP = CO x SVR.[2]

You will frequently encounter the MAP = CO x SVR equation throughout this book. Remember, this is not a straightforward calculation; you cannot just feed in numbers from various machines. The units here do not neatly align. It is more of a conceptual tool than an exact mathematical formula, so I think it is "accurate-ish." Delving too deeply into its physiological and sophisticated aspects would deviate from the purpose of this book, which is to provide a practical, bedside approach. For a more in-depth analysis, there are other texts dedicated to that.

The MAP = CO x SVR equation evolves from a more intricate formula: MAP = (Preload x Afterload)/Resistance. It is easier to conceptualize this equation using values obtained through hemodynamic monitoring devices (such as pulmonary artery catheters, pulse-contour analysis, and bioreactance) or echocardiography.

As a quick refresher: Preload is the volume of blood in the heart's ventricles at the end of diastole, the heart's relaxation phase. The 'tank' must be adequately filled to maintain the optimal preload. Think of afterload as the resistance the heart contends with during blood ejection—too high, and the heart labors; too low, it is akin to lifting featherweight dumbbells. It is that straightforward. In this context, resistance refers to the opposition faced by blood as it flows through the circulatory system.

Understanding Hemodynamic Parameters: A Focus on MAP, CO, and SVR
In critical care, the nuanced understanding of hemodynamic parameters is pivotal. Among these, the equation MAP = CO x SVR forms the cornerstone. Let's delve into what each component signifies and why they are crucial in managing patients, especially when using vasopressors and inotropes.

Mean Arterial Pressure (MAP): More Than Just a Number
What does MAP truly represent in critical care? MAP, or mean arterial pressure, is often the go-to metric for assessing patient status. We were all trained that MAP

13

was calculated using the formulas MAP = DBP + 1/3(SBP − DBP) or MAP = DBP + 1/3(PP). However, in hospitals, we rely more on oscillometric devices for these measurements, which accurately determine MAP but algorithmically estimate systolic and diastolic pressures.[3-5] This method can lead to discrepancies compared in the SBP and DBP, versus with direct measurements, like those from an arterial line. Generally speaking, oscillometric and arterial line MAPs correlate.

Clinically, a MAP of 65 mmHg is considered adequate for resuscitation, as per the *Surviving Sepsis Campaign* guidelines.[6] However, focusing solely on MAP can be misleading. Understanding the effects of vasopressors and inotropes on cardiac output (CO) and systemic vascular resistance (SVR) is crucial. Over-reliance on MAP can overshadow the importance of a balanced management approach.

Cardiac Output (CO): The Heart of the Matter
Cardiac output is the heart's minute-by-minute performance, measured in liters per minute (L/min). It is the product of heart rate (HR) and stroke volume (SV).[7] SV, in turn, is the volume ejected by the left ventricle per beat, influenced by preload, contractility, and afterload. Notably, SV can also be further broken down into left ventricular end-diastolic and end-systolic volumes, revealing the intricate dynamics of cardiac function.

Systemic Vascular Resistance (SVR): The Circulatory Challenge
SVR represents the resistance faced by blood within the circulatory system. It is a function of vascular tone, vessel diameter, and blood viscosity. Traditionally calculated as (MAP - right atrial pressure)/CO,[2] SVR is typically measured in dynes s/cm$_5$, though Wood units (mL/L/min) are also utilized. It is vital to understand that SVR is more complex than a mere indicator of left ventricular afterload,[8] yet we often equate the two for simplicity. As Voltaire said, "Perfect is the enemy of good"—a principle that applies well to this simplification for better comprehension.

Central Venous Pressure (CVP): A Component on the Sidelines
CVP, measured in the superior vena cava or right atrium, reflects the pressure in the central venous system.[9] While it incorporates elements like blood volume and cardiac function, its normal value is close to zero,[10] rendering it less significant in the MAP = CO x SVR equation.

Applying these Concepts
Let us consider a patient with septic shock. They arrive at the emergency department with a suspected infection. The urinalysis suggests a urinary source. The standard procedure involves fluid resuscitation, antibiotics, labs, and initiating norepinephrine. However, what if the patient does not respond as expected, even with escalating vasopressors? This scenario underscores the importance of evaluating CO. In cases of potential sepsis-induced cardiomyopathy, with an incidence of 20%,[25] an excessive focus on increasing

SVR can be counterproductive if CO is compromised. Thus, considering all aspects of hemodynamic stability, a multi-pronged approach is essential for optimal patient care.

What is a vasopressor?
In the complex arena of critical care, understanding the role of vasopressors is crucial for managing conditions like distributive shock. By inducing vasoconstriction, vasopressors play a pivotal role in countering vasodilation, restoring blood pressure, and ensuring adequate organ perfusion. When we consider the MAP = CO x SVR equation, vasopressors primarily act to enhance SVR, thereby increasing MAP.

However, it is vital to recognize that more is not always better. While increasing SVR is beneficial up to a point, excessive vasoconstriction can backfire by overly increasing cardiac afterload. This can inadvertently compromise CO, the very function we aim to support. This delicate balance underscores the preference for norepinephrine in many clinical scenarios. Norepinephrine's α effects promote vasoconstriction, enhancing SVR, while its β effects support CO, offering a more balanced hemodynamic profile.

Contrary to common bedside terminology, not all 'vasopressors' are solely vasoconstrictive. Medications like norepinephrine, epinephrine, and dopamine, often labeled as vasopressors, are more accurately described as 'inoconstrictors.' These drugs possess both inotropic (affecting the force of cardiac contraction) and vasoconstrictive properties. This dual action makes them unique and distinct from pure vasopressors such as phenylephrine, vasopressin, angiotensin II, and midodrine.

What is an inotrope?
Inotropes are medications that increase the heart's contractile force, akin to how spinach boosts Popeye's strength. They enhance the heart's ability to pump blood more effectively. Within the MAP = CO x SVR equation context, inotropes primarily improve CO by influencing the contractility aspect of SV and, to varying degrees, the HR. In this text, we focus on positive inotropes, which increase contractility, as opposed to negative inotropes, which are outside the scope of this book.

What are inodilators?
While inotropes are straightforward in their action on contractility, we often encounter medications that do more in clinical practice. Inodilators, such as milrinone and dobutamine (sometimes), not only enhance contractility but also dilate blood vessels. This dual action means they improve CO but can also decrease SVR, potentially exacerbating hypotension. This double effect places them in a unique category within the inotrope family.

What are inoconstrictors?
Inoconstrictors, including norepinephrine, epinephrine, and dopamine, act on both β receptors (inotropic effect) and α receptors (vasopressor effect). They increase both CO and SVR, thereby improving MAP effectively. This dual action makes them particularly valuable in specific clinical scenarios where a balance of enhanced contractility and vasoconstriction is needed.

THE RECEPTORS
Understanding the intricate roles of the receptors is pivotal in grasping how vasopressors and inotropes influence the MAP = CO x SVR equation. This knowledge is crucial, especially in treating and managing critically ill patients. Let's journey to demystify these receptors, highlighting their impact in critical care settings. Attempts have been made to make this content enjoyable, a fool's errand. I would not blame you for skipping this section on your first read and using it as a reference as you power through the rest of the book. How about just glossing over it rather than skipping it?

Alpha (α) receptors
The α receptors, also known as α-adrenergic receptors, found throughout the body, play a key role in our body's fight or flight responses. These receptors are divided into two main subtypes: α-1 and α-2, each with its unique role in critical care. Vasopressors that act on the α receptors described in this book include norepinephrine, epinephrine, phenylephrine, dopamine, and, to a lesser extent, dobutamine.[12]

Alpha-1 receptors (α-1): Located primarily in the smooth muscle of blood vessels, the α-1 receptors, especially the α-1B subtype, are central in managing vasoconstriction. When discussing α-1 receptors in this book, it is usually the α-1B we refer to, given its crucial role in increasing SVR in the MAP equation. Meanwhile, α-1A receptors, predominantly found in the prostate and bladder, are often targeted in treating conditions like benign prostatic hyperplasia (BPH). This explains the urinary retention observed in many septic shock patients. The effects of activating the α-1D receptors are less understood. Interestingly, α-1D receptors are the predominant α-1 receptor subtype in the epicardial coronary arteries.[13]

Alpha-2 receptors (α-2): These are fascinatingly diverse in their location and function. In the brain, they can have sedative and anxiolytic effects. In the heart, their role is more subtle, affecting heart rate and contractility. The β receptors overshadow it. In the adrenal glands, activation of the α-2 receptors inhibits the release of norepinephrine, resulting in negative feedback regulation of sympathetic activity. This can result in vasodilation and reduced blood pressure. Their involvement in pain and inflammation regulation also makes them significant in critical care.

Beta (β) receptors

Beta receptors, known scientifically as β-adrenergic receptors, are pivotal in the intricate symphony of the human body's response mechanisms. Located on the surface of cells in various tissues and organs, these receptors play crucial roles in physiological and pharmacological processes. They are classified into three main subtypes: β-1, β-2, and β-3, each with distinct locations and functions, underscoring their clinical significance.

Beta-1 receptors (β-1): The β-1 receptors are primarily located in the heart and play a significant role in regulating cardiac output. Activation of β-1 receptors leads to increased heart rate (positive chronotropic effect), increased myocardial contractility (positive inotropic effect), and increased conduction velocity through the atrioventricular (AV) node. Beyond the heart, β-1 receptors in the kidneys aid in renin release, a hormone pivotal for blood pressure regulation. In the liver, they facilitate glycogenolysis, a process crucial for maintaining blood glucose levels.

Beta-2 receptors (β-2): Primarily located in the smooth muscle cells of the bronchi, blood vessels, and uterus, β-2 receptors have diverse roles. Activation of β-2 receptors in the lungs results in bronchodilation, helping to relieve bronchospasm. In the uterus, β-2 activation helps play a role in relaxing the smooth muscle. They also increase lipolysis in fat cells, which releases free fatty acids into the bloodstream. β-2 activation also leads to increased muscle and liver glycogen breakdown and enhanced glucose release from the liver.

Beta-3 receptors (β-3): These are mainly in the brown adipose tissue (fat cells) and the urinary bladder. Activation of β-3 receptors in adipose tissue promotes lipolysis (the breakdown of fat) and can have thermogenic effects. The thermogenic effects come from the breaking down of fat, causing heat. In the urinary bladder, β-3 receptor activation relaxes the detrusor muscle, which can improve bladder emptying. β-3 receptors are also found in the heart, regulating heart rate and contractility.

Dopaminergic Receptors

Dopaminergic receptors are pivotal in the brain's neurotransmission, responding to dopamine, a versatile neurotransmitter and vasopressor. These receptors are categorized into two main families: the D1-like receptors (D1 and D5) and the D2-like receptors (D2, D3, and D4).[21] The dopamine stocked at our hospital binds to the D1 and D2 receptors, although some literature says it also binds to the D4 receptors.[22]

D1-like Receptors: In the context of dopamine's role as a vasopressor, these receptors, particularly in the renal vasculature, are implicated in modulating blood flow and sodium excretion, influencing blood pressure regulation.[23] The D1-like receptors, coupled with Gs proteins, increase cyclic AMP (cAMP) levels in neurons, generally eliciting excitatory responses. They are involved in regulating motor control and reward processing and are abundant in regions like the striatum. Data suggests that the D1 dopaminergic receptors can be found in the cerebral, coronary, mesenteric, and renal vasculature, platelets, and lymphocytes.[24]

D2-like Receptors: These are coupled with Gi proteins, leading to reduced cAMP levels and typically producing inhibitory effects. These receptors are integral in modulating mood, cognition, and behavior and are targeted by antipsychotic medications. When acting as a vasopressor, dopamine also interacts with D2-like receptors in the peripheral vasculature. Here, dopamine's action can lead to vasodilation or vasoconstriction, depending on the receptor subtype and the vascular bed involved.

The numerous functions of dopaminergic receptors throughout the brain and body are beyond the book's scope. A separate book can be written about the dopaminergic receptors, given the different types and locations of each of these. Given the limited use cases of dopamine today, I recommend alternative sources for deeper explanations.

Vasopressin Receptors
Vasopressin receptors, essential in various physiological processes, are classified into two primary types: V1 and V2. The V1 receptor has two subtypes, V1a and V1b, sometimes referred to in literature as vasopressin type 1A, V1A, and V1a.

V1a Receptors: These receptors are primarily located in vascular smooth muscle cells, where they induce vasoconstriction and muscle contraction.[14] An intriguing aspect of V1a receptors is their involvement in myocardial hypertrophy, evidenced by increased V1a mRNA in vascular smooth muscle.[15] Their presence is notable in several organ systems. In the kidneys, V1a receptors in mesangial cells, efferent arterioles, and renal tubules enhance water reabsorption, thus reducing urine output and increasing blood volume. In the liver, activation of these receptors leads to glycogenolysis in hepatocytes. V1a receptors are also found in blood components like leukocytes, stimulating chemotaxis, chemokine production, and antibody production. Their role in inducing platelet aggregation is clinically significant, especially in the context of vasopressin's effects. In the brain, V1a receptors influence behavior, cortisol synthesis and secretion, and the regulation of circadian rhythms.

V1b Receptors: These receptors are predominantly in the anterior pituitary gland and pancreas.[14] They are instrumental in stimulating ACTH secretion in the brain.[15] Meanwhile, in the pancreas, their activation is linked to glucagon release, regulation of intracellular Ca2+ levels, and cellular proliferation.

V2 Receptors: These receptors are found on the renal tubular cells, specifically on the basolateral surface.[14] They are vital in water reabsorption and central to the

18

anti-diuretic hormone (ADH) function. In the kidneys, V2 receptor activation impacts several areas, including the macula densa, intermediate, distal, and collector tubules. These effects extend to signal transduction, AQP2 shuttling to the cell surface for water permeability, AQP2 mRNA synthesis, and the regulation of intracellular cAMP.

Contrary to the effects on V1a receptors, V2 receptor stimulation leads to vasodilation. These receptors also contribute to bone remodeling and have anti-inflammatory effects in the lungs.[15] An essential function of V2 receptors is the induction of von Willebrand factor secretion,[16] which clarifies the effectiveness of DDAVP in treating uncontrolled bleeding in patients with uremia.

Angiotensin Receptors
Angiotensin receptors are part of the renin-angiotensin system, significantly regulating blood pressure, fluid balance, and SVR.

Angiotensin II Type 1 Receptors (AT1):   These receptors are the most common and are primarily responsible for the well-known actions of angiotensin II. They are widely distributed in various tissues, including the vascular smooth muscle, heart, kidneys, brain, and adrenal glands. Activation of AT1 receptors leads to vasoconstriction, increased blood pressure, aldosterone secretion, sodium retention, and potassium excretion. They also stimulate the release of antidiuretic hormone (ADH) and facilitate sympathetic nervous system activity. AT1 receptors are the primary target of angiotensin receptor blockers (ARBs), a class of drugs utilized to treat hypertension, heart failure, and diabetic nephropathy. This receptor target for *Giapreza* (Angiotensin II) will be discussed in a later chapter.

Angiotensin II Type 2 Receptors (AT2): These receptors are less understood than AT1. They are found in many tissues, including the heart, kidneys, adrenal glands, brain, and fetal tissues. The AT2 receptor is believed to counter-regulate the effects of the AT1 receptor, potentially mediating vasodilation and promoting cell differentiation and tissue repair. However, the physiological and pathophysiological roles of AT2 receptors are still being researched.

Understanding Clinical Trial Phases
Understanding the distinct objectives of each phase in clinical trials is crucial for appreciating new treatments' development and evaluation process.

Phase I Trials: The primary goal of Phase I trials is to assess the safety of a potential treatment. This initial phase focuses on determining the appropriate dosage range and identifying side effects. These trials, conducted with a small group of participants, lay the groundwork for further testing by establishing basic safety parameters. They are not meant to change our practice.

Phase II Trials: These trials delve into the efficacy of the treatment. The aim is to evaluate whether the treatment produces the desired effect in the target condition. While still involving a relatively small participant group, these trials provide preliminary data on the treatment's effectiveness and further safety evaluation. Trials in this phase are also not intended to change practice.

Phase III Trials: These are the practice-changing trials. In Phase III, the treatment is compared against the current standard of care. This phase involves a larger participant group, often spanning multiple locations, to thoroughly assess the treatment's effectiveness, monitor side effects, and collect more comprehensive safety data. Phase III trials are pivotal in determining whether the treatment is effective and safe enough to be considered for approval by regulatory bodies.

Phase IV Trials: After a treatment receives regulatory approval, Phase IV trials are conducted. These post-marketing studies aim to understand the treatment's long-term effects and benefits in a broader population. They also continue monitoring for adverse reactions or side effects over extended use.

Cardiac Surgery-Related Vasoplegia
Cardiac surgery involving cardiopulmonary bypass (CPB) can induce a systemic inflammatory response in some patients, leading to profound vasodilation. This condition is referred to here as cardiac surgery-related vasoplegia for consistency. Defining cardiac surgery-related vasoplegia precisely remains a challenge within the medical community. Clinically, these patients often emerge from surgery with significantly low SVR, typically in the range of 400-700 dynes s/cm$_5$, as opposed to the normal (depending on the source) range of 800-1200 dynes s/cm$_5$. They are usually already on vasopressors, with their CO elevated due to the drastically reduced SVR. Their heart faces minimal afterload. Upon ICU admission post-surgery, the anesthesiologist often preps the team for a potential 'battle,' ranging from a short skirmish to a prolonged multi-day war.

When discussing the patient's condition with families, I simplify the explanation by likening it to an allergic reaction to the pump, as blood contact with the tubing can trigger this response. A key focus is on pre-surgery medication history, particularly the use of β-blockers, calcium channel blockers (CCBs), angiotensin-converting enzyme (ACE) inhibitors, or angiotensin receptor blockers (ARBs), as these can be risk factors for vasoplegia.[17] Adherence to medication regimens, sometimes leading to unintended pre-surgery consumption of these drugs, is a common issue. Additional risk factors include prolonged duration on CPB and a low ejection fraction, with arginine vasopressin deficiency also playing a role.[18] The incidence of vasoplegia ranges between 5-25%.[19] This book will discuss the treatment options for cardiac surgery-related vasoplegia.

Without trying to provoke additional confusion, different names for this pathology include cardiac surgery-related vasoplegia, vasoplegia syndrome, vasoplegia syndrome after cardiac surgery, vasoplegic syndrome, post-cardiothoracic surgery, post-cardiac surgery vasoplegia, and post-cardiotomy vasoplegia. For the sake of standardization in this text, I have selected 'cardiac surgery-related vasoplegia' as the terminology for this book.

Norepinephrine-Equivalent Dosing

Norepinephrine-equivalent dosing (NED) has emerged in the literature to compare different vasopressor dosages. The benefit of establishing a NED would allow us to level the playing field in clinical trials. In the supplementary text of the ATHOS-3 trial, we can find the following NED: 0.1 µg/kg/min of norepinephrine is equal to 0.1 µg/kg/min of epinephrine, 15 µg/kg/min of dopamine, 1 µg/kg/min of phenylephrine, and 0.4 U/min of vasopressin.[20] There will be occasions when this term arises in subsequent chapters.

Citations

eddyjoemd.com/the-basics-citations

02: NOREPINEPHRINE

Let's kick off with norepinephrine—the go-to vasopressor for most physicians—as 97% of physicians prefer it as the first choice in managing septic shock.[1] Suppose a patient crashes, and you cannot determine the underlying cause. In this situation, norepinephrine is an excellent bandaid to provide time to figure out the etiology. Aligning with this approach, the *Surviving Sepsis Campaign* emphatically endorses norepinephrine as the first line, recommending it over other alternatives.[2]

What is the mechanism of action of norepinephrine?
Norepinephrine—with dual roles as a neurotransmitter and hormone—mainly targets α and β-adrenergic receptors throughout the body. However, it has a more pronounced impact on α receptors than on β receptors. Here, we explore both aspects.

When norepinephrine activates α-1 receptors on smooth muscle cells, it causes vasoconstriction, substantially increasing systemic vascular resistance (SVR) and contributing to the rise in mean arterial pressure (MAP). Additionally, its interaction with α-2 receptors impedes further norepinephrine release from presynaptic neurons, serving as a negative feedback mechanism. Other physiological implications of α-2 receptor agonism extend beyond the critical care scope.[3] Regarding β receptors, norepinephrine's engagement with β-1 receptors increases heart rate (HR) and contractility, thus maintaining or enhancing cardiac output (CO).[10,11] However, the relationship with β-2 receptors remains somewhat vague. While some studies exhibit negligible β-2 activity,[4,5] others propose some level of involvement.[6-9]

The concept of Ventriculo-Arterial (V-A) coupling sheds light on how norepinephrine further improves SV and CO.[26,27] This concept involves stimulating both α and β receptors to synchronize the heart to enhance contractility. Moreover, α receptor stimulation increases coronary perfusion pressure and the arterial system afterload, enhancing ventricular contractility. V-A coupling increases SV when these α effects are integrated with the known β effects on contractility.

In clinical practice, several studies have demonstrated improvements in cardiac parameters due to norepinephrine, including increased CO and systemic venous oxygen saturation (SvO2),[12] an elevated cardiac index and stroke volume index,[13] a higher cardiac index,[14] and an increase in SV.[26]

At what dose should we start norepinephrine?

According to the package insert, the recommended initial dose for norepinephrine is 8-12 µg/min, with subsequent titration based on patient response.[15] However, in my experience across various institutions, the more common practice is to initiate treatment at lower doses. This conservative approach allows for cautious monitoring and adjustment according to the patient's specific requirements and responses.

What is the half-life of norepinephrine?

Norepinephrine has a relatively short half-life of approximately 2.4 minutes.[15] This is in stark contrast to vasopressin, which has a longer half-life of 10 to 35 minutes.[16] Understanding the differences in half-lives between norepinephrine and vasopressin, especially when strategizing vasopressor weaning. More details on this perspective will be discussed in the upcoming sections.

How high can we crank up the norepinephrine?

The highest recorded norepinephrine dose in medical literature was administered to a 36-year-old man at a staggering 30 µg/kg/min.[17] In this case, the team continued to increase the dosage as long as the patient's MAP responded positively. Remarkably, this aggressive approach helped the patient survive. However, it is essential to note that numerous studies have linked high doses of norepinephrine to increased mortality rates.[18-21] For instance, one study concluded that doses exceeding 1.0 µg/kg/min were associated with a 90% mortality rate,[19] while another reported an 83% mortality rate at similar doses.[18] Nonetheless, these high mortality rates are not surprising, considering that such high doses are typically administered to critically ill patients who might otherwise not survive at all.

In conditions like septic shock, where mortality rates vary between 20 and 30% depending on the study,[22-24] the use of high-dose norepinephrine might be justified in particular situations. Despite the risks, exceeding traditional dose limits could save 10 to 17% of patients.[18,19] From my experience, careful consideration, judicious use, and informed consent in potentially salvageable cases are imperative. It is essential to weigh the potential benefits against the underlying risks like gut and digital ischemia. The hard maximum doses typically utilized by many institutions deserve further deliberation and assessment. In some cases, these risks might be non-trivial. However, the alternative option is certain death.

Should we use weight-based or non-weight-based dosing for norepinephrine?

The choice between weight-based dosing (WBD) and non-WBD for norepinephrine is a topic of ongoing debate. In my case, I have always worked in environments where non-WBD is the norm. Therefore, I am not familiarized with interpreting WBD measurements like 'xxx µg/kg/min.' However, despite my inclination towards non-WBD, I acknowledge the potential precision of WBD. But what does the research indicate?

First, it is essential to note that direct comparisons between WBD and non-WBD are scarce. The few existing studies on this topic are limited in scope and methodology, often being retrospective.[27,28] One key finding is that WBD and non-WBD accomplish a similar MAP after initiation, regardless of the patient's body mass index (BMI). Remarkably, in a study with about 30% obese patients, those in the WBD group needed a smaller norepinephrine dose to reach the required MAP and had a lower total norepinephrine utilization. However, a significant observation was that 27% of patients in the WBD group necessitated continuous renal replacement therapy (CRRT), compared to just 12% in the non-WBD group, a statistically significant difference (p=0.01).[28] However, the study's retrospective nature leaves us looking for reasons for this discrepancy to be clarified.

Another noticeable point is that obese patients with WBD received higher cumulative doses of norepinephrine and experienced a longer weaning period.[27] Given the existing data and its limitations, the superiority of one method over the other cannot be conclusively established.

When is the optimal time to start norepinephrine in septic shock?
According to the *Surviving Sepsis Campaign*, norepinephrine should be initiated in cases of persistent hypotension despite adequate fluid resuscitation.[2] However, the exact timing and the amount of fluid resuscitation necessary before initiating vasopressors are still subjects of ongoing studies.

In a retrospective study, Waechter *et al.* identified a 'sweet spot' for initiating vasopressors between 1 and 6 hours after the onset of septic shock.[29] Although the statistical techniques utilized in this research are complex, the findings are remarkable. Another retrospective study indicated that initiating norepinephrine after six hours from diagnosis resulted in a doubled mortality rate, suggesting that starting vasopressors within six hours is preferable.[30]

However, a *post hoc* analysis of the ARISE trial data, which investigated early goal-directed therapy in sepsis, suggested that early vasopressor usage might be associated with higher 90-day mortality.[31] This finding offers a contrasting perspective to the earlier studies. As a quick reminder, the ARISE trial was among the three trials published between 2014 and 2015, evaluating early goal-directed therapy versus standard care in sepsis.[24]

More recent data from the CENSER trial in 2019 demonstrated that initiating norepinephrine within a median of 93 minutes of arrival at the emergency department (compared to 3 hours and 12 minutes in standard therapy) had significant benefits.[32] These benefits included a higher percentage of patients reaching the targeted MAP and organ perfusion goal by 6 hours (76.1% vs. 48.4%, p < 0.001) and others, such as reduced cardiogenic pulmonary edema and fewer arrhythmias. Although there was no statistically significant difference in 28-day mortality (15.5% vs. 21.9%, p=0.15), the trial was not powered to validate this endpoint.

In their 2020 comprehensive analysis, Ospina-Tascon *et al.* utilized a prospectively collected database to evaluate the outcomes of 186 septic shock patients. These individuals were propensity-matched based on the timing of vasopressor administration.[33] The study classified patients into two groups: those who received vasopressors either before or within one hour of fluid resuscitation (termed the Very Early Vasopressor group, or VE-VP) and those who received vasopressors after an hour following fluid resuscitation (termed the Delayed Vasopressor group, or D-VP). The findings from this study were illuminating. The VE-VP group — receiving vasopressors more promptly — exhibited multiple advantages. Notably, they required less cumulative resuscitation fluids compared to the D-VP group.

The reduced fluid requirement also resulted in a lower net fluid balance for the VE-VP group. Most significantly, the study reported a marked difference in mortality rates between the two groups. For instance, the VE-VP group had a considerably lower mortality rate at 18.3%, in contrast to the D-VP group's 38.7% (p=0.03). A common concern in managing septic shock is the potential for under-resuscitation, leading to adverse effects such as acute kidney injury or ischemic digits. The analysis did not observe these adverse effects in the VE-VP group. This finding implies that when balanced with appropriate fluid resuscitation, early vasopressor administration can be safe and beneficial in improving patient outcomes.

In summary, a meta-analysis including these studies leans towards early initiation of norepinephrine. It has several benefits, such as a shorter time to reach the target MAP, reduced IV fluid requirements within six hours, and potentially associated with decreased mortality.[34] Nonetheless, further large-scale trials are needed to solidify these findings.

In cases of septic shock with low cardiac output, should we use norepinephrine and dobutamine or epinephrine alone?
Managing septic shock, particularly along with Sepsis-Induced Cardiomyopathy (SIC), which recent data suggests has a prevalence of about 20%,[35] requires careful use of a vasopressor strategy. Our typical approach involves initiating norepinephrine and adding vasopressin as the second-line agent in septic shock. However, this scenario can lead to suboptimal treatment in one in five patients if SIC is not identified and addressed suitably. It is vital to implement mechanisms for identifying SIC to customize treatment accordingly. Therefore, a pivotal

26

question is whether to add dobutamine to norepinephrine or to switch to epinephrine in such scenarios.

The 2007 CATS trial offers some insights into this dilemma. It illustrated no significant difference in various outcomes between patients treated with either epinephrine (alone or combined with dobutamine) and norepinephrine for septic shock patients with low cardiac index.[36] Although the study observed more frequent transient elevations in lactate levels in the epinephrine group, there were no notable differences in the rate of serious adverse effects.

Given that norepinephrine is the recommended first-line vasopressor in septic shock patients, according to the *Surviving Sepsis Campaign*, adding dobutamine to an already-running norepinephrine infusion has a practical advantage. This approach minimizes waste and simplifies management. However, the potential drawback could be limited IV access or pump availability for managing two distinct infusions. Thus, the choice between adding dobutamine or switching to epinephrine should be based on clinical efficacy and practical logistics in each patient's unique situation.

Is this combination of norepinephrine and dobutamine superior to epinephrine non-AMI cardiogenic shock?

A randomized controlled trial (RCT) conducted in 2011 sheds light on this question. In this study, 30 patients with non-acute myocardial infarction (AMI) cardiogenic shock were randomized to receive either epinephrine alone or a combination of norepinephrine and dobutamine.[37] These patients were meticulously managed using a pulmonary artery catheter, a crucial step given the risk of exacerbating cardiac stress with excessive afterload.

The trial revealed multiple transient but significant effects in patients receiving epinephrine. These included an increase in HR, a rise in lactate levels at 12 hours, an increase in gastric hypoperfusion, and a greater insulin requirement. The significance of the lactate increase—explored in the *Epinephrine* chapter—is not currently thought to have a substantial clinical impact. However, these findings led the authors to conclude that combining norepinephrine and dobutamine was more reliable and safer than epinephrine for managing non-AMI cardiogenic shock. Given the complexities of cardiac management in shock states, this study highlights the importance of a tailored approach, favoring the combined use of norepinephrine and dobutamine over epinephrine in specific non-AMI cardiogenic shock scenarios.

In cases of cardiogenic shock following a myocardial infarction, is norepinephrine superior to epinephrine?

Intuitively, one may assume epinephrine to be more beneficial in acute myocardial infarction (AMI) cases due to its potent β action, which theoretically should enhance CO. However, the findings from the OptimaCC study challenge this assumption.[5]

The OptimaCC study was a double-blind pilot study designed to compare norepinephrine with epinephrine in patients experiencing cardiogenic shock secondary to an AMI.[5] Unfortunately, the study was halted prematurely after the enrollment of only 57 patients. Despite being underpowered and thus not statistically significant, the results raised serious concerns: 48% of patients in the epinephrine group did not survive, compared to 27% in the norepinephrine group. Moreover, refractory shock was observed in 37% of the epinephrine group, whereas it was much lower at 7% in the norepinephrine group (p=0.008). Although the confidence intervals were wide, these safety issues were significant enough to discontinue the trial.

As anticipated, the epinephrine group exhibited transiently higher heart rates and increased lactate levels. These findings imply that norepinephrine might be safer and more effective than epinephrine in managing cardiogenic shock post-AMI, contrary to past assumptions.

When did norepinephrine replace dopamine as the preferred vasopressor in the ICU?
The pivotal change in ICU vasopressor preference from dopamine to norepinephrine can be traced back to the findings of the SOAP II trial in 2010. This RCT involved 1679 shock patients who were administered either dopamine or norepinephrine as their first-line vasopressor for shock.[38]

The study illustrated various trends implying a potential mortality benefit with norepinephrine. However, these findings did not reach statistical significance. Moreover, the higher incidence of arrhythmias in patients receiving dopamine significantly influenced the clinical preference. In the trial, approximately a quarter of the patients (24.1%) treated with dopamine developed arrhythmias, compared to only 12.4% in the norepinephrine group—a statistically significant difference (p < 0.001).

This marked difference in the incidence of arrhythmias played a crucial role in steering clinical practice towards favoring norepinephrine over dopamine as the first-line vasopressor in the ICU setting.

How does norepinephrine compare to dopamine in the treatment of cardiogenic shock?
The SOAP II trial also significantly impacted the debate between norepinephrine and dopamine in cardiogenic shock patients in 2010.[38] This trial included patients with various types of shock (hypovolemic, septic, and cardiogenic) and randomized them to receive either dopamine or norepinephrine.[38] Notably, the

subgroup with cardiogenic shock demonstrated the worst outcomes when treated with dopamine.

Further cementing the case against dopamine was a systematic review and meta-analysis published in 2017. This analysis incorporated data from nine studies and highlighted a higher mortality rate associated with the use of dopamine in cardiogenic shock. Moreover, it reported a lower risk of arrhythmia with norepinephrine.[39]

The bottom line from these findings was quite clear: the use of dopamine in cardiogenic shock patients has little to no justification, especially when compared to norepinephrine. This evidence has gradually shifted the clinical preference towards norepinephrine as the more effective and safer choice in managing cardiogenic shock.

Is there truth to the adage '*Levophed*, leave 'em dead'?
This phrase—often heard in clinical practice and training—typically refers to concerns about increased mortality or the risk of ischemia in different body parts due to the use of norepinephrine (*Levophed*). However, a closer look at the data offers a more nuanced understanding.

A systematic review and meta-analysis clarified this issue, as it found that peripheral ischemia—a significant concern with vasopressors—occurs in approximately 3.13% of patients treated with norepinephrine.[41] Interestingly, dopamine was specified as having a higher risk, with digital ischemia developing in 6.53% of patients. When considering the risk of AMI, the occurrence was similar in patients on norepinephrine (3.03%) and those on epinephrine (3.11%). As for arrhythmias, they were most commonly observed in 8.33% of patients on norepinephrine. Once again, dopamine presented a higher risk, with arrhythmias noted in 26.01% of patients. These findings indicated that while norepinephrine carries certain risks, such as peripheral ischemia and arrhythmias, its adverse effect profile is not as severe as dopamine.

Therefore, the '*Levophed, leave 'em dead*' adage represents more of a myth than a reflection of clinical reality, especially while considering the comparative risks associated with other vasopressors.

In septic shock patients with baseline atrial fibrillation, should we opt for norepinephrine or phenylephrine?
The decision between norepinephrine and phenylephrine in septic shock patients with atrial fibrillation hinges on the different receptor targets of these drugs. For instance, phenylephrine—acting solely on α receptors—is often favored, assuming it evades exacerbating cardiac stress through β effects, unlike norepinephrine.

A retrospective study involving 1847 patients with atrial fibrillation and receiving norepinephrine or phenylephrine provides valuable insights.[42] Some patients also received rhythm and rate control medications, including amiodarone, β-blockers, and digoxin. The key outcome of this study was that patients on phenylephrine had a slightly lower HR than those on norepinephrine. The difference was modest, averaging just four beats per minute less, encompassing patients with and without rapid ventricular rate (RVR). More specifically, in the RVR cohort, the HR was six beats per minute lower on average in the phenylephrine group, a difference that was statistically significant but not clinically impressive. Additionally, the two groups had an insignificant difference between the conversion rates to sinus rhythm (p=0.7) and mortality (p=0.9).

These findings suggest that while phenylephrine may modestly reduce HR compared to norepinephrine in septic shock patients with atrial fibrillation, the clinical significance of this difference may be limited. Therefore, choosing between these two vasopressors should consider other patient factors and treatment goals.

If a septic shock patient develops atrial fibrillation with RVR, should we switch from norepinephrine to phenylephrine?
This question was the focus of a retrospective study involving 67 septic shock patients. They were first treated with norepinephrine and subsequently developed atrial fibrillation with RVR.[43] The study compared patients who continued on norepinephrine with those who were switched to phenylephrine, evaluating their outcomes in achieving sustained rate control.

The findings revealed that switching to phenylephrine did not significantly improve the primary endpoint of sustained rate control compared to continuing norepinephrine. However, the authors noted that their finding "*suggests a potential clinical effect on achieving rate control*" with phenylephrine. While this study does not conclusively advocate for switching to phenylephrine in such cases, it hints at a potential benefit in rate control.

Should norepinephrine also be the first-line vasopressor in cardiac surgery-related vasoplegia?
This question was evaluated in the VANCS trial—an RCT comparing norepinephrine with vasopressin in managing cardiac surgery-related vasoplegia.[44] This trial is also discussed in the *Vasopressin* chapter. Involving 300 patients, the study evaluated the occurrence of a composite primary outcome, which included mortality or severe complications, in both treatment groups.

The results were significant: the composite outcome occurred in 32% of patients in the vasopressin group, compared to 49% in the norepinephrine group (p=0.0014). Severe complications were specifically defined as stroke, the need for mechanical ventilation for over 48 hours, deep sternal wound infection, the necessity for reoperation, or acute renal failure.

In the VANCS trial, the dosage ranges for the vasopressors were noteworthy. Norepinephrine was administered between 10 to 60 µg/min, whereas vasopressin was titrated from 0.01 to 0.06 U/min. Another key finding was the lower incidence of atrial fibrillation in the vasopressin group. Based on these outcomes, the authors concluded that vasopressin might be more suitable as the first-line vasopressor in patients with vasoplegic shock after cardiac surgery.

In which cases should norepinephrine not be the first-line vasopressor?
Patients with hypotension or shock secondary to hypertrophic obstructive cardiomyopathy should avoid norepinephrine as the initial vasopressor.[45] Similarly, patients exhibiting systolic anterior motion (SAM) of the mitral leaflet are advised against norepinephrine.[46] In these scenarios, norepinephrine administration, which increases contractility and systemic vascular resistance, may worsen left ventricular outflow tract obstruction, thereby impairing hemodynamics.[54]

Vasopressors lacking β receptor activity are preferable for aortic or mitral valve stenosis patients. Phenylephrine is often recommended as the first-line treatment for hypotension in cases of aortic stenosis.[46] Furthermore, the American Heart Association (AHA) recommends using phenylephrine or vasopressin as the first-line treatment for cardiogenic shock resulting from mitral stenosis.[47]

Does norepinephrine cause immunosuppression?
The relationship between norepinephrine and the immune system, particularly in sepsis, is complex and not fully understood. Sepsis triggers a multifaceted immune response, where both pro-inflammatory and anti-inflammatory responses can become dysregulated.[48] The concern is whether norepinephrine—a commonly utilized vasopressor in sepsis management—might contribute to this dysregulation, possibly leading to immunoparalysis.

This concern was highlighted in research by Stolk *et al.*, which discussed how α-adrenergic and β-adrenergic receptor activity of norepinephrine might impact immune responses.[49] The study concluded that α-adrenergic stimulation can increase pro-inflammatory cytokine production, such as TNF-α, IL-6, and IL-1β. On the other hand, β-adrenergic stimulation appeared to have the opposite impact, decreasing these pro-inflammatory cytokines but increasing IL-10, which has anti-inflammatory and immunosuppressive properties.[50] Only *in vitro* and animal *in vivo* studies had been published then.[49]

Further expanding on these findings, Stolk *et al.* conducted a study in 2020 that evaluated the immunomodulating effects in human subjects.[51] The authors adopted a comprehensive approach, first evaluating the immunologic effects *in vitro* using primary human leukocytes, followed by murine models, and finally, exploring the effects in humans *in vivo*. Their findings suggest that norepinephrine can indeed dysregulate the host response to sepsis.

These revelations raise critical questions for clinicians. For example, given its lack of similar immunoparalysis effects, should we consider initiating vasopressin earlier in treating septic shock patients? Furthermore, there might be no imminent study on the horizon as per a recent search on clinicaltrials.gov. Thus, understanding the full impact of norepinephrine on immune function in septic patients is a critical area for future exploration.

FUN FACTS!

Discovery of Norepinephrine: Norepinephrine was first discovered in 1947 by Ulf von Euler, an achievement that earned him the Nobel Prize in 1970.[52]

Clinical Trials Initiation: Human clinical trials seem to have started around 1953.[53]

FDA Approval: 1950.[15]

Alternate Names for Norepinephrine: Nor-adrenaline, noradrenaline, Levaterenol, Levophed, Arterenol, noradrenaline tartrate, and noradrenaline acid tartrate.

Are All Norepinephrine Formulations the Same? Leone *et al.* highlighted in a letter that there could be significant differences in the interpretation of guideline recommendations for norepinephrine dosing, depending on whether the patient is receiving norepinephrine base or norepinephrine tartrate.[55] This discrepancy underscores the need for a consensus on dosing standards, which is still unresolved.

Citations

eddyjoemd.com/norepinephrine-citations

03: EPINEPHRINE

Epinephrine is probably the first vasopressor we learned about, thanks to its prominent role in movies like Quentin Tarantino's 'Pulp Fiction' and 'Crank' featuring Jason Statham. It is a medication that often gets dramatically called for in every cardiac arrest scene on television. While it remains our primary choice for patients in cardiac arrest, its use in other etiologies of shock has diminished.

What is the mechanism of action of epinephrine?
Similar to norepinephrine, epinephrine also targets the α-1, α-2, β-1, and β-2 adrenergic receptors. As discussed in *The Basics* chapter, activation of α-1 adrenergic receptors results in vasoconstriction in both arterial and venous circuits, leading to increased systemic vascular resistance (SVR). Stimulating β-1 receptors produces positive inotropic and chronotropic effects, increasing cardiac output (CO) through elevated heart rate (HR) and stroke volume (SV). These contribute to an increase in the mean arterial pressure (MAP).

In the equation MAP = CO x SVR, epinephrine elevates CO (via HR and contractility) and SVR. It might seem like the ultimate go-to vasopressor since it covers all bases. Review articles and books often compare the receptor binding of norepinephrine and epinephrine because they activate the same receptors.

Many have traditionally understood that norepinephrine exhibits a higher affinity for α receptors, while epinephrine leans toward β receptor binding. However, the extent of receptor activation is not an exact science. While there is a consensus that epinephrine boasts superior β activity compared to norepinephrine, peer-reviewed literature reveals variations in α and β receptor binding.
• Epinephrine and norepinephrine have equal α-1 affinity.[1-7]
• Epinephrine has less α affinity than norepinephrine.[8,9]

There are variations even amongst the effect distribution of epinephrine itself.
• Epinephrine has more β affinity than α affinity.[1,5,8,10,11]
• Epinephrine has the same β affinity as α. [2,3,7]

These variations underscore the complexity of epinephrine's pharmacodynamics, reminding us that critical care medicine still holds many areas for deeper understanding. Beyond vasoconstriction and cardiac effects, epinephrine's stimulation of β-2 receptors leads to bronchodilation and glycogenolysis. The latter process involves the conversion of glycogen to glucose in the liver and skeletal muscles, which contributes to elevated lactate levels—a topic that will be discussed in more detail later.

Is the function of epinephrine dose-dependent?

Epinephrine's function varies depending on the dose, which initially surprised me, and you may find it new information too. It is a learning curve for all of us, especially since many review articles on vasopressors only sometimes delve into these dose-dependent effects.[2,3,5,6,12]

At lower doses, epinephrine primarily acts as an inotrope by activating β-1 adrenergic receptors, thereby increasing CO.[10,13] Surprisingly, SVR tends to decrease at these lower doses. Therefore, in the MAP = CO x SVR equation, a rise in CO coupled with a decrease in SVR could result in no significant change in MAP. The definition of 'low-dose' epinephrine varies, with some literature citing > 4 µg/min[14] and 2-10 µg/min[8] for non-weight-based, and < 0.01 µg/kg/min[10] or 0.01 to 0.1 µg/kg/min[8] for weight-based dosing.

Conversely, epinephrine's effects on α-1 receptors become more prominent at higher doses than its β receptor effects.[7,9,14] This leads to an increase in both CO and SVR, resulting in an elevated MAP. The definition of 'high-dose' epinephrine also varies, with some sources defining it as 0.05-0.5 µg/kg/min,[10] > 1.0 µg/kg/min,[10] or simply any dosage exceeding the 'low-dose' range.[7,14] These varying definitions highlight the complexity of epinephrine dosing and its impact on hemodynamics. Understanding these nuances is vital to optimizing its use in clinical settings.

Why is epinephrine not the first-line vasopressor in shock?

The 2008 CAT study significantly influenced Epinephrine's role as a first-line vasopressor in shock, a randomized controlled trial (RCT) comparing epinephrine and norepinephrine in treating various shock etiologies.[15] This study enrolled 280 patients, and while there were no significant differences in hemodynamic responses between the two groups, the epinephrine arm experienced a higher incidence of adverse effects.

Notably, patients receiving epinephrine developed tachycardia and an increase in lactate levels. Although these effects were transient, resolving after 24 hours, the elevated lactate levels caused enough concern for some patients to be withdrawn from the study by their treating clinicians. This concern over adverse effects, particularly the transient rise in lactate, led to a shift in clinical practice patterns. As a result, norepinephrine became the preferred first-line vasopressor in managing shock.

Why do we no longer use epinephrine in cardiogenic shock?

The rationale against using epinephrine in cardiogenic shock has been established for over a decade. At first glance, epinephrine seems ideal for cardiogenic shock due to its β-1 adrenergic stimulation, which enhances both HR and SV, thereby improving CO. However, this apparent benefit comes with a significant drawback: the increase in myocardial oxygen consumption at the cellular level.[15] This increased myocardial oxygen demand can be detrimental, especially in patients with cardiogenic shock, whose hearts are already compromised. The increased oxygen consumption exacerbates the risk of ischemia and arrhythmias, essentially overstraining the heart.[17] This concern is supported by soon-to-be-discussed studies leading to a consensus in the medical community to avoid epinephrine in managing cardiogenic shock.

Is this combination of norepinephrine and dobutamine superior to epinephrine non-AMI cardiogenic shock?
An RCT conducted in 2011 sheds light on this question. In this study, 30 patients with non-AMI cardiogenic shock were randomized to receive either epinephrine alone or a combination of norepinephrine and dobutamine.[17] These patients were meticulously managed using a pulmonary artery catheter, a crucial step given the risk of exacerbating cardiac stress with excessive afterload.

The trial revealed several transient but significant effects in patients receiving epinephrine. These included an increase in HR, a rise in lactate levels at 12 hours, an increase in gastric hypoperfusion, and a greater insulin requirement. The significance of the lactate increase, which will be explored later in the epinephrine chapter, is not currently thought to have a substantial clinical impact. However, these findings led the authors to conclude that combining norepinephrine and dobutamine was more reliable and safer than epinephrine for managing non-AMI cardiogenic shock. Given the intricacies of cardiac management in shock states, this study highlights the importance of a tailored approach, favoring the combined use of norepinephrine and dobutamine over epinephrine in specific non-AMI cardiogenic shock scenarios.

In cases of cardiogenic shock following a myocardial infarction, is epinephrine superior to norepinephrine?
Intuitively, one might assume epinephrine to be more beneficial in acute myocardial infarction (AMI) cases due to its potent β action, which theoretically should enhance CO. However, the findings from the OptimaCC study challenge this assumption.[5]

As discussed in the *Norepinephrine* chapter, The OptimaCC study was a double-blind pilot study designed to compare norepinephrine with epinephrine in patients experiencing cardiogenic shock secondary to an AMI.[4] Unfortunately, the study had to be halted prematurely after enrolling only 57 patients. Despite being underpowered and thus not statistically significant, the results raised serious concerns: 48% of patients in the epinephrine group did not survive, compared to 27% in the norepinephrine group. Furthermore, refractory shock was observed in 37% of the epinephrine group, whereas it was much lower at 7% in the norepinephrine group (p=0.008). Although the confidence intervals were wide, these safety issues were significant enough to discontinue the trial.

As anticipated, the epinephrine group exhibited transiently higher heart rates and increased lactate levels. These findings suggest that norepinephrine might be safer and more effective than epinephrine in managing cardiogenic shock post-AMI, contrary to previous assumptions.

In a 2018 meta-analysis of 16 studies to find the relationship between epinephrine and short-term survival of 2583 patients, there was a higher risk of death in the epinephrine cohort than in other regimens.[18] These data had numerous limitations best described by the authors, including limited prospective RCTs. However, compared to other drug therapies, epinephrine had a threefold increase in mortality risk. To wrap up the discussion, given the current data, epinephrine has been taken out of the game as the American Heart Association has named norepinephrine as the vasopressor of choice for cardiogenic shock.[3]

In cases of septic shock with low cardiac output, should we use norepinephrine and dobutamine or epinephrine alone?
Managing septic shock, particularly when accompanied by sepsis-induced cardiomyopathy (SIC), which recent data suggests has a prevalence of about 20%,[19] requires careful consideration of vasopressor strategy. Our usual approach involves initiating norepinephrine and adding vasopressin as the second-line agent in septic shock. However, this could lead to suboptimal treatment in one in five patients if SIC is not identified and addressed appropriately. It is crucial to implement mechanisms for identifying SIC to tailor treatment accordingly. The pivotal question then becomes whether to add dobutamine to norepinephrine or to switch to epinephrine in these situations.

The 2007 CATS trial provides some insights into this dilemma. It demonstrated no significant difference in various outcomes between patients treated with either epinephrine alone or a combination of dobutamine and norepinephrine for septic shock with low cardiac index.[20] However, the study observed more frequent transient elevations in lactate levels in the epinephrine group, with no notable differences in the rate of serious adverse effects or overall efficacy.

Given that norepinephrine is the recommended first-line vasopressor in septic shock, according to the *Surviving Sepsis Campaign*, there is a practical advantage to adding dobutamine to an already-running norepinephrine infusion. This approach minimizes waste and simplifies management. The potential drawback, however, could be limited IV access or pump availability for managing two separate infusions. Thus, the choice between adding dobutamine or switching to epinephrine should be made considering both clinical efficacy and practical logistics in each patient's unique context.

When could epinephrine be the first-line vasopressor in septic shock?
Epinephrine may be considered as the first-line vasopressor in septic shock under specific circumstances, particularly in resource-limited settings. The

Surviving Sepsis Campaign has acknowledged the high cost of norepinephrine in developing countries,[12] leading to the more frequent use of epinephrine as a cost-effective alternative.[21] Additionally, the CATS trial highlighted situations where patients with refractory shock and myocardial dysfunction might benefit from epinephrine. In such cases, epinephrine can be utilized as a standalone treatment or combined with norepinephrine and dobutamine.[20]

What are the adverse effects of epinephrine?
These include increased HR, leading to tachyarrhythmias. Additionally, epinephrine can decrease regional blood flow, causing splanchnic vasoconstriction and mesenteric ischemia.[36] Another notable adverse effect is the elevation of lactate levels, which can complicate the clinical picture and management.[12,22] Cardiac toxicity has been reported from prolonged and high doses of epinephrine.[1]

Why does epinephrine cause an elevation in lactate?
There is a common misperception that elevated lactate levels are synonymous with sepsis. While the *Surviving Sepsis Campaign* recommends checking lactate levels in suspected sepsis cases,[12] it is crucial to recognize that lactate elevation has a broad differential diagnosis.[23] This has also led to the coined term *"Lacto-Bolo reflex"* by Dr. Rory Spiegel, where clinicians reflexively order fluid boluses for elevated lactate levels.[24] However, elevated lactate is not always indicative of tissue hypoxia. Sepsis is often more about enhanced aerobic glycolysis in skeletal muscle than tissue hypoxia.[26]

The physiological mechanisms behind lactate production, particularly concerning epinephrine use, are complex but essential to understand. Repeat after me: *"Lactate is not the boogeyman. Lactate is not always a marker of tissue hypoxia."*.[25] Exogenous and endogenous epinephrine stimulates β-2 adrenergic receptors, enhancing aerobic glycolysis in skeletal muscle cells.[15,20,26,27] This process leads to increased glucose production, which is metabolized to pyruvate. Pyruvate then faces a crossroad: it can either be metabolized into Acetyl CoA via pyruvate dehydrogenase (PDH), leading to the Krebs cycle and substantial (38) ATP production, or it can follow the lactate pathway, which is less efficient in terms of ATP production (only 2) but still serves as a fuel source for the brain and heart.[29] Under conditions of increased glycolysis and adrenergic stimulation, PDH can become, shall we say, overwhelmed. This leads to a diversion of pyruvate into the less efficient lactate pathway.[30] This is exacerbated in sepsis, which inhibits PDH, further increasing lactate production.[20] It is important to understand that this lactate production is not pathologic or a result of tissue hypoxia.

In summary, while epinephrine does raise serum lactate levels, this increase is not necessarily harmful.[15-17,20,27,28] Clinicians should be cautious about relying solely on trending lactate levels during resuscitation in patients receiving epinephrine and may instead consider using capillary refill testing as a more appropriate measure.[31]

How long can we expect the elevated lactate to last?
The elevation in lactate levels observed with epinephrine administration is typically transient, with normalization expected within 24 hours. This timeframe for lactate normalization has been documented in two separate trials.[15,20] It is important to note that this reduction in lactate levels occurs naturally, without the need for interventions such as fluid administration to 'dilute' the lactate.

Is combining epinephrine and dobutamine synergistic?
Combining epinephrine and dobutamine, based on their mechanisms of action, might seem like it would lead to a synergistic improvement in CO. However, this is not the case, as per the findings of a 1998 study.[32] The expected additive effect of these two drugs in enhancing CO was not observed in the cardiac surgery population. Instead, the authors described the interaction between epinephrine and dobutamine as a 'pseudoantagonism.'

This unexpected result suggests that combining epinephrine and dobutamine does not necessarily enhance therapeutic outcomes and may require careful monitoring for hemodynamic and cardiovascular effects. While this specific finding pertains to the cardiac surgery population, it raises questions about the efficacy of this combination in other forms of cardiogenic shock. However, thorough studies in these areas are lacking.

What is the highest dose of epinephrine in the literature?
In the context of epinephrine dosing, the package insert suggests an infusion rate ranging from 0.05 µg/kg/min to 2 µg/kg/min.[34] However, higher doses have been documented in clinical research and practice. For instance, the CATS trial administered epinephrine at 5-60 µg/kg/min,[12] significantly exceeding the package insert's recommendations. The term 'refractory shock' in the literature is often associated with epinephrine doses higher than 0.5 µg/kg/min.[33] However, it is crucial to recognize that there is no universally defined maximum dose for epinephrine in cases of refractory shock.[8] This lack of a definitive upper limit indicates the need for individualized dosing based on patient response and the severity of their condition, underscoring the importance of clinical judgment and continuous monitoring in managing such critical scenarios.

FUN FACTS!

First Adrenal Medullary Hormone Identified: Epinephrine is the first hormone identified from the adrenal medulla.
Discovery: John Jacob Abel in 1897.[35]
FDA Approval: 1939.[34]

Citations: eddyjoemd.com/epinephrine-citations

04: PHENYLEPHRINE

Poor phenylephrine. It is the weakest of the vasopressors.[1] To achieve a predetermined MAP, phenylephrine doses could be 220% higher than norepinephrine. We tend to reach for it as a third or fourth vasopressor in cases of septic shock, only to watch the dose quickly climb in minutes. We will explore several scenarios where phenylephrine could be a game-changer and save some lives.

What is the mechanism of action of phenylephrine?
Phenylephrine acts selectively on the α1-adrenergic receptors, specifically targeting the α-1A, α-1B, and α-1D subtypes. The α-1A and α-1B receptors are predominantly in peripheral blood vessels, where phenylephrine's action affects arterial and venous tone.[3] This action increases systemic vascular resistance (SVR), increasing the mean arterial pressure (MAP) in the equation MAP = CO x SVR. No effect is noted on the cardiac output (CO).

However, phenylephrine's interaction with the α-1D receptors, primarily found in the epicardial coronary arteries, could result in coronary vasoconstriction.[4] This is an important consideration in patients with coronary artery disease.

Unlike some other vasopressors, phenylephrine does not act on the β-adrenergic receptors.[5] This specificity means that while it increases SVR, it could decrease CO due to the increased afterload and/or reflex bradycardia, a compensatory mechanism of the body in response to the increased vascular resistance.[6]

When was phenylephrine first considered as a treatment option for septic shock?
The exploration of phenylephrine as a potential treatment for septic shock began after norepinephrine had been extensively studied in this context. Researchers were particularly concerned about ensuring that the increase in peripheral resistance induced by phenylephrine did not lead to significant adverse effects. One central area of focus was the potential for gut ischemia, a concern raised due to norepinephrine's known effect of decreasing mesenteric blood flow.[2]

In 2008, a pilot study was conducted to assess the impact of phenylephrine on patients with septic shock, employing advanced monitoring techniques such as gastric tonometry and thermo-dye dilution catheter, pulmonary artery catheter, and radial artery catheters.[2] This study involved just 14 patients initially treated with norepinephrine, switched to phenylephrine for 8 hours, and then reverted to norepinephrine. Extensive hemodynamic parameters and laboratory values were measured during these phases.

The results of this study, however, were somewhat disheartening. The data indicated that phenylephrine led to a decrease in hepatosplanchnic blood flow and impaired renal function. These findings raised concerns about the suitability of phenylephrine in the management of septic shock, particularly in terms of its impact on vital organ perfusion.

What did we learn from the first RCT of phenylephrine in septic shock?

The first randomized controlled trial (RCT) comparing phenylephrine to norepinephrine in septic shock, published in 2008, came shortly after the pilot study discussed earlier and interestingly involved many of the same researchers.[1] This study was conducted against the backdrop of the *Surviving Sepsis Campaign's* 2008 recommendations, which listed norepinephrine or dopamine as the preferred first-line vasopressors.[7]

In this RCT, 32 patients with septic shock were randomized to receive either phenylephrine or norepinephrine for 12 hours.[1] A significant aspect of this study was its response to previous concerns about phenylephrine's impact on splanchnic blood flow. Utilizing sophisticated measurement techniques similar to the pilot study, the researchers did not observe the same reduction in hepatosplanchnic blood flow or impairment in renal function that had been noted earlier. Moreover, the study did not find the expected decrease in cardiac index, which could have been caused by excessive afterload (SVR), nor did it observe reflex bradycardia.

While these results did not demonstrate the superiority of phenylephrine over norepinephrine, they did suggest that phenylephrine could be a safe alternative in treating septic shock, according to the data from this particular study. In my opinion, this study is too small and limited in duration to translate to daily patient management in the ICU.

Why is phenylephrine not considered a first-line vasopressor in sepsis?

The reliance on RCTs for guiding management in critical care is standard, but sometimes, real-world circumstances, like drug shortages, inadvertently influence clinical practice. A notable example was the national norepinephrine shortage from February 2011 to February 2012, which compelled clinicians to use alternative vasopressors for septic shock.[8]

A retrospective analysis from a 26-hospital database examined whether there was an association between the norepinephrine shortage and increased mortality in septic shock.[8] It was observed that the use of phenylephrine in septic shock patients rose significantly, from 36.2% to 54.4%, the highest increase among the alternative vasopressors. Concurrently, in-hospital mortality in septic shock patients increased from 35.9% to 39.6%.

This rise in mortality led to discussions and debates within the medical community, with some clinicians attributing the increase directly to phenylephrine. However, others pointed out that the causes could be multifactorial, noting the limitations of retrospective data.[9-11] Additionally, the use of other vasopressors like dopamine and vasopressin also increased significantly during this period, raising questions about the sole culpability of phenylephrine.

While norepinephrine is established as a superior vasopressor for septic shock, the assignment of blame to phenylephrine for the observed increase in mortality may be overstated. If we were to hypothetically attribute the 3.7% increase in mortality solely to phenylephrine, it would result in a number needed to harm (NNH) of 27, meaning that treating 27 patients with phenylephrine could potentially harm one. However, this NNH is likely an overestimation, and the actual number could be much higher, given the complexities and multifactorial nature of septic shock management.

What does the *Surviving Sepsis Campaign* say about using phenylephrine in septic shock?
As of the 2021 *Surviving Sepsis Campaign* Guidelines, phenylephrine is not mentioned.[12] This omission contrasts with previous guidelines, where phenylephrine was recommended only in specific situations. These included cases of high-cardiac output septic shock as a salvage therapy option or in scenarios where norepinephrine was found to induce serious arrhythmias.[13,14]

In septic shock patients with baseline atrial fibrillation, should we opt for norepinephrine or phenylephrine?
The decision between norepinephrine and phenylephrine in septic shock patients who also experience atrial fibrillation hinges on the different receptor targets of these drugs. Phenylephrine, acting solely on α receptors, is often favored, assuming it avoids exacerbating cardiac stress through β effects, unlike norepinephrine.

A study involving 1847 patients with atrial fibrillation, who were either started on norepinephrine or phenylephrine, provides valuable insights.[11] It is important to note that some patients also received rhythm and rate control medications, including amiodarone, β-blockers, and digoxin.

The key finding of this analysis was that patients on phenylephrine had a slightly lower heart rate than those on norepinephrine. The difference was modest, averaging just four beats per minute less, encompassing patients with and without rapid ventricular rate (RVR). Specifically, in the RVR cohort, the heart rate was, on average, six beats per minute lower in the phenylephrine group, a difference that was statistically significant but not clinically impressive.

Additionally, there was no significant difference in the rates of conversion to sinus rhythm (p=0.7) nor in mortality (p=0.9) between the two groups.

These findings suggest that while phenylephrine may modestly reduce HR compared to norepinephrine in septic shock patients with atrial fibrillation, the clinical significance of this difference may be limited. Thus, when choosing between these two vasopressors, clinicians should consider other patient factors and treatment goals.

If a septic shock patient develops atrial fibrillation with RVR, should we switch from norepinephrine to phenylephrine?
This question was the focus of a retrospective study involving 67 septic shock patients who were initially treated with norepinephrine and subsequently developed atrial fibrillation with RVR.[10] The study compared patients who continued on norepinephrine with those who were switched to phenylephrine, analyzing their outcomes in achieving sustained rate control.

The findings revealed that switching to phenylephrine did not significantly improve the primary endpoint of sustained rate control compared to continuing norepinephrine. However, the authors noted that their data "suggests a potential clinical effect on achieving rate control" with phenylephrine. While this study does not definitively advocate for switching to phenylephrine in such cases, it hints at a possible advantage in rate control.

Should we use phenylephrine as the second-line vasopressor?
The current standard of care typically involves adding vasopressin as the second-line vasopressor for patients with septic shock.[12] The question then arises: what if phenylephrine was utilized instead? Unfortunately, prospective data is lacking to answer this question.

Our most relevant study is a retrospective analysis comparing the outcomes of patients who received vasopressin versus phenylephrine as a second-line vasopressor, in addition to norepinephrine.[9] This study included 287 patients, and notably, 57% of the patients in the phenylephrine group were treated before 2011, a period before vasopressin was commonly utilized.

Despite the expectation that advancements in sepsis management over the years would have negatively impacted the outcomes for the phenylephrine group, the study found no significant difference in ICU mortality, hospital mortality, the need for renal replacement therapy, or the lengths of stay in the ICU and hospital. These findings were unexpected, as one might anticipate worse outcomes with phenylephrine than vasopressin.

However, it is essential to approach these results with caution due to the inherent limitations of retrospective studies. While the findings do not show phenylephrine in a negative light compared to vasopressin, prospective studies would be necessary to form a more definitive conclusion regarding the efficacy of phenylephrine as a second-line vasopressor in septic shock. It also does not make logical sense to continue targeting the same α-receptors that norepinephrine is already activating.

Why is phenylephrine particularly useful in HOCM?

Hypertrophic obstructive cardiomyopathy (HOCM) is characterized by an obstruction in the left ventricular outflow tract (LVOT) due to a thickened heart septum. This obstruction limits blood flow from the left ventricle to the aorta, creating a fixed blood flow dynamic. In HOCM, increased heart workload—through higher heart rate or contractility—exacerbates this obstruction by increasing the pressure gradient, known as a dynamic gradient, across the LVOT. This can be life-threatening, potentially leading to cardiac arrest if the gradient becomes excessively high. Vasopressors that increase heart rate and contractility, particularly those with β-adrenergic activity, could worsen this situation.

Phenylephrine, with its α-adrenergic effects, becomes valuable in this context. It increases systemic vascular resistance (SVR) and, consequently, the afterload on the heart.[28] This increase in afterload helps to expand the cross-sectional area of the LVOT, reducing the dynamic gradient during systole.[5] Using standard vasopressors with β-adrenergic activity and inotropes in HOCM could inadvertently heighten the LVOT obstruction and harm patients.

Historically, methoxamine, an α-1 agonist, was demonstrated to increase the LVOT diameter in patients with HOCM in a study conducted in 1964.[16] Reflecting this understanding, both the American College of Cardiology Foundation/ American Heart Association in 2011 and the European Society of Cardiology in 2014 have included phenylephrine in their guidelines for treating hypotension in HOCM, especially in cases unresponsive to fluid therapy.[17,18]

Why is phenylephrine recommended for hypotensive patients with aortic stenosis?

Phenylephrine is often the first-line treatment for patients experiencing hypotension in the context of aortic stenosis.[3] Patients with aortic stenosis are characterized by having a fixed maximum CO due to the obstructed blood flow from the left ventricle. This fixed output means that medications that increase HR or contractility through β-adrenergic effects could be detrimental, mainly if they induce arrhythmias.

An advantageous aspect of using phenylephrine in these patients is its ability to increase coronary perfusion pressure and induce reflex bradycardia. While typically considered an adverse effect in other contexts, reflex bradycardia can be beneficial in aortic stenosis. It helps to reduce myocardial oxygen consumption, alleviating the stress on the heart. This effect makes phenylephrine a safer choice compared to vasopressors with β-adrenergic activity.

Supporting this approach, a small study demonstrated that the administration of phenylephrine did not adversely affect left ventricular performance in patients with aortic stenosis.[19] This finding suggests that phenylephrine can be safely utilized in this patient group without compromising cardiac function.

Is phenylephrine recommended for patients with mitral stenosis?
The American Heart Association recommends using phenylephrine or vasopressin in cases of cardiogenic shock secondary to mitral stenosis.[20] This recommendation is particularly relevant in scenarios where definitive treatment is the ultimate goal, but there is an immediate need to stabilize the patient.

Cardiogenic shock in the context of mitral stenosis is often characterized as a preload-dependent state. Optimizing diastolic filling time is critical, which can be achieved by slowing the heart rate. In this situation, inotropes or vasopressors that exert β-adrenergic effects are generally not advisable, as they are unlikely to improve hemodynamics.

Due to its action on α-adrenergic receptors without β-adrenergic effects, phenylephrine becomes a suitable choice. Its use can help manage the hemodynamic challenges in mitral stenosis by maintaining vascular tone without increasing the heart rate. This approach can be critical in ensuring adequate cardiac filling and maintaining systemic perfusion until more definitive interventions can be implemented.

Why is phenylephrine commonly used as a push-dose vasopressor?
Push-dose vasopressors have become increasingly popular in acute medical scenarios where immediate intervention is necessary and standard vasopressor infusions are not readily available. This situation often arises in medical wards or emergency settings where a patient is deteriorating rapidly, and moving them to the ICU immediately is not feasible.

Phenylephrine is a convenient choice for push-dose administration due to its pharmacokinetic properties. It has a rapid onset of action, typically around one minute, comparable to epinephrine and norepinephrine.[21] However, its duration of action, lasting between 10 and 20 minutes, is notably longer than that of norepinephrine, which lasts only 1 to 2 minutes. This extended duration is a significant advantage in emergencies. It provides a critical window for healthcare staff to prepare and initiate more sustainable vasopressor infusions, including the time needed for pharmacy coordination, pump setup, and tubing priming.

The caveat with push-dose vasopressors, including phenylephrine, is the limited robust data supporting their use.[22] Conducting RCTs in such urgent and ethically sensitive scenarios presents considerable challenges, as the necessity for immediate life-saving interventions often precludes the feasibility of traditional research methodologies. "Oh, hello, Mr. Crashing Patient. We are conducting an RCT on push-dose vasopressors. By signing here, you consent to receive either life-sustaining vasopressors now or a placebo". Patient arrests.

Should we administer a push-dose of phenylephrine to unstable septic shock patients before starting norepinephrine?
In emergencies where septic shock patients remain hypotensive despite fluid resuscitation and there's a delay in starting peripheral vasopressor infusions, push-dose vasopressors like phenylephrine can be considered as a stopgap measure. This approach is often contemplated to stabilize hemodynamics quickly.

A study by a team at the Cleveland Clinic provides some insight into this practice.[23] They analyzed data from 141 patients who received a phenylephrine push (1000 µg syringes at 100 µg/mL concentration) before vasopressor infusion. They compared them to 282 patients who did not receive such a push. The study found that achieving hemodynamic stability at 3 hours was more likely with push-dose phenylephrine. However, a notable finding was the higher ICU mortality in the phenylephrine push group (31.2% vs. 22%). The authors speculated that this increased mortality might be linked to the cardiac effects of phenylephrine.

However, it is important to interpret these findings cautiously. In the critical scenario of a patient rapidly deteriorating from septic shock, the immediate priority is to restore adequate perfusion. The use of push-dose vasopressors can be a vital intervention in such cases. It is challenging to attribute the higher mortality solely to the use of push-dose phenylephrine, as these patients might already be in a more severe condition, necessitating immediate intervention.

This study highlights the importance of considering potential confounders in database research. In emergencies, medications are often administered urgently, with documentation and ordering potentially delayed. These factors, not accounted for in the study, could impact the interpretation of the results. I'm not going to allow my patient to remain unstable and hypotensive while chasing down the norepinephrine infusion because of the results of this paper.

The study underscores why reading the article yourself is crucial rather than relying solely on abstracts or summaries (or even this book). In practice, the decision to use push-dose vasopressors, including phenylephrine, should be based on the immediate clinical needs of the patient and the available resources while acknowledging the limitations and potential biases of existing research.

Is phenylephrine helpful in managing cardiac surgery-related vasoplegia?

Norepinephrine and vasopressin are the most extensively studied and recommended for treating cardiac surgery-related vasoplegia.[24] While some experts suggest limiting the use of phenylephrine in this context,[25] its application may be necessary in certain challenging cases.

Patients with refractory cardiac surgery-related vasoplegia, where standard treatment options are inadequate, often require individualized management based on their specific hemodynamic profiles. In these scenarios, phenylephrine can be a viable option, especially when an increase in SVR is warranted without the additional β-adrenergic effects that other vasopressors might provide.

Can patients on phenylephrine be switched to midodrine?

Transitioning patients from phenylephrine to midodrine is a viable strategy, considering both drugs share a similar mechanism of action. This approach was explored in a 2013 observational trial conducted in a surgical ICU setting.[26] In this trial, patients on stable phenylephrine doses were switched to midodrine. The findings indicated that introducing midodrine facilitated a quicker weaning of phenylephrine. This is particularly relevant in the context of transitioning patients from the ICU, where phenylephrine is administered intravenously, to oral medications like midodrine as they stabilize and move toward recovery.

What adverse effects should be vigilant about in clinical practice?

One of the most clinically significant adverse effects to monitor for is bradycardia, which has been recognized since as early as 1942.[27] This effect is often attributed to the activation of pressure receptors located in the carotid sinus and aortic arch, leading to what is sometimes referred to as baroreceptor mediated reflex bradycardia.[6]

Bradycardia can have substantial implications for patient management, especially if it negatively impacts the MAP in the MAP = CO x SVR equation. In such cases, the reduced CO caused by the slowed heart rate might counteract the benefits of increased SVR, diminishing overall hemodynamic stability.

FUN FACTS!

Patent Year: 1934.[3]

First Human Studies: The first studies involving phenylephrine in humans were conducted in 1942.[27]

Alternate Names: Phenylephrine is known by several other names, including Biorphen, Vazculep, and IMMPHENTIV. While these names might be less familiar, phenylephrine is often called neosynephrine, Neo-synephrin, or simply "Neo" in clinical settings.

Citations: eddyjoemd.com/phenylephrine-citations

05: VASOPRESSIN

Vasopressin is our second favorite vasopressor after norepinephrine. It is the number one backup dancer to norepinephrine's killer (no pun intended) moves. After all, epidemiological data demonstrates that vasopressin is prescribed to 17.2% of patients in septic shock.[1] Per those data, I say "backup dancer," as vasopressin is only the first-line vasopressor in 6.1% of performances. In 93.9% of the time, it performs alongside other vasopressors. One could consider it like when Jennifer Lopez and Britney Spears married their backup dancers. Am I mentioning J.Lo and Britney in a critical care medicine book? I should stop rambling now.

What is the mechanism of action of vasopressin?
Vasopressin binds to three receptor subtypes: V1a, V1b, and V2.[2] Regarding hemodynamics, vasopressin primarily increases the mean arterial pressure (MAP) by increasing the systemic vascular resistance (SVR) in the MAP = CO x SVR equation. Increases in cardiac output (CO) are not generally noted with vasopressin. The functions of these receptors are described in far more detail in *The Basics* chapter.

Why do septic shock patients develop intrinsic vasopressin insufficiency?
As vasopressin is an endogenously produced hormone, our bodies bolster production should we need more, like in sepsis, right? Well... no. Multiple postulated mechanisms exist to ascertain why it does not work as we wish, and we, unfortunately, end up with a vasopressin deficit.
- **Baroreflex-Mediated Secretion:** Vasopressin secretion is primarily regulated by baroreflex mechanisms. When hypovolemia and hypotension occur, vasopressin release should increase and flex its anti-diuretic muscles. On the contrary, when adequately hydrated, stretch receptors in the left atrium, aortic arch, and carotid sinus inhibit vasopressin secretion.[3] Unfortunately, its response is often limited in septic shock.
- **Initial Surge and Subsequent Decline:** Early in septic shock, vasopressin levels can surge as the body's response to stress. However, these levels tend to taper off over time.[4] Sepsis can increase nitric oxide production, contributing to vasodilation and further inhibiting vasopressin production. In addition, endogenous and exogenous norepinephrine may inhibit the release of endogenous vasopressin.[3]
- **Depletion of Vasopressin Stores:** MRI studies of septic shock patients have demonstrated a complete depletion of vasopressin stores in the neurohypophysis, leaving insufficient vasopressin available for an impactful response.[5] We do not have enough endogenous vasopressin to go into battle with a realistic chance of winning. The lead author of the VASST trial has aptly noted that "*Vasopressin should be thought of as replacement therapy for relative deficiency rather than as a vasopressor agent to be titrated to effect.*"[6]

47

What about patients with cardiac surgery-related vasoplegia?
The endogenous vasopressin deficiency observed in septic shock patients also appears in patients who develop cardiac surgery-related vasoplegia. In this case, vasopressin levels have been demonstrated to be even lower than the expected normal response for the degree of hypotension.[7,8] Comparatively, vasopressin levels were even lower in this patient population than in septic shock patients.[8] If your patient suffers from cardiac surgery-related vasoplegia, adding vasopressin makes sense. There will be more on this topic in the forthcoming sections.

Is this same intrinsic vasopressin insufficiency observed in cardiogenic shock?
No, intrinsic vasopressin insufficiency is not typically observed in cardiogenic shock. A study has demonstrated that patients in cardiogenic shock tend to maintain appropriate intrinsic plasma vasopressin levels. For instance, the mean intrinsic plasma level of vasopressor in septic shock patients was 3.1 pg/mL.[4] Cardiogenic shock patients, however, had a mean intrinsic plasma vasopressin level of 22.7 pg/mL, which was considered appropriate. While many patients may initially preserve their SVR, cardiogenic shock patients can deteriorate and experience vasodilation if not treated promptly, leading to a distinct clinical presentation.

Does vasopressin increase the blood pressure in normotensive patients?
Vasopressin may not substantially increase blood pressure in normotensive patients.[9,10] Clinical studies involving healthy volunteers have demonstrated minimal blood pressure increases in response to vasopressin infusions, just 5-7 mmHg.[9] The cardiovascular reflex systems in normotensive individuals appear to buffer the vasopressor effect of vasopressin. This information reinforces that vasopressin may not significantly affect blood pressure when normotensive patients receive it. The claim that vasopressin loses its effect when a patient is normotensive appears accurate. This could also explain why vasopressin does not need to be weaned — more on weaning in subsequent sections.

Once started, when will the vasopressin infusion kick in?
Vasopressin behaves differently than catecholamine vasopressors in terms of onset of action. While catecholamines like norepinephrine exhibit rapid effects, vasopressin takes longer to take full effect. The peak effect of a vasopressin infusion is typically achieved within 15 minutes, with the effect diminishing approximately 20 minutes after discontinuation, considering its half-life of 10-35 minutes.[2]

What was observed in the first clinical trials of vasopressin?
It is wild to contemplate that the early clinical trials exploring vasopressin in septic shock took place during our lifetimes (mostly), dating back to the late 1990s and early 2000s.[4,11-13] These studies included small groups of septic shock patients who received variable vasopressin doses. The trials primarily aimed to

explore whether vasopressin could serve as a catecholamine-sparing vasopressor. In 1997, a small group of patients in septic shock were evaluated, where the researchers experimented with doses of 0.01 U/min and 0.04 U/min.[4] Interestingly, 6 out of 10 patients got off their first-line catecholamine vasopressor. Due to the success of that first trial, a 1999 trial including ten septic shock patients observed its efficacy in refractory septic shock. The authors utilized 0.04 U/min of vasopressin versus placebo.[11]

The first randomized controlled trial (RCT) comparing vasopressin to norepinephrine in 24 septic shock patients was published in 2002.[12] Both vasopressin and norepinephrine were titrated over 4 hours while reaching doses of 0.08 U/min in the vasopressin group and 16 µg/min in the norepinephrine group. The catecholamine-sparing effects were again observed. The size of the trials grew with a 2003 study enrolling 48 patients who were already on norepinephrine to remain on that dose or receive the combination of norepinephrine and vasopressin so many of us utilize today.[13] After this study, the floodgates opened with more robust data being published.

What are the must-know trials involving vasopressin?
Several landmark trials have significantly shaped our understanding of vasopressin's role in septic shock:

VASST (VAsopressin vs. Norepinephrine in Septic Shock STudy)
In 2008, the VASST trial made significant strides in our understanding of vasopressin's role in septic shock management.[6] It was an RCT that compared the combination of vasopressin and norepinephrine with norepinephrine alone as the primary vasopressor. Notably, the study utilized a vasopressin dose range of 0.01-0.03 U/min, aiming to address the physiological deficiency of vasopressin in this patient population. In contrast, the norepinephrine dose ranged from 5-15 µg/min. It is noteworthy that patients were not initially randomized to vasopressin but instead initiated on norepinephrine and subsequently transitioned to vasopressin.

The VASST trial was conducted and published within a decade of the first pilot study of vasopressin in septic shock. This reflects the rapid progression of our knowledge. The VASST trial enrolled 778 patients. Upon its conclusion, the trial did not reveal statistically significant differences in 28-day mortality (39.3% with vasopressin vs. 35.4% with norepinephrine, $p = 0.26$) or 90-day mortality (43.9% vs. 49.6%, $p = 0.11$). There were no differences in adverse effects.

While the overall results demonstrated no marked differences in mortality, a critical observation emerged when scrutinizing a specific patient subgroup. Those categorized as experiencing "*less severe septic shock*" — defined as requiring less than 15 µg/min of norepinephrine at randomization — exhibited a significant reduction in mortality when treated with vasopressin. The 28-day mortality number needed to treat (NNT) was 10.9 (26.5% vs. 35.7%, $p=0.05$), and the 90-

day mortality NNT was 9.7 (35.8% vs. 46.1%, p=0.04). These findings painted a more favorable picture, indicating a notable benefit for patients with less severe septic shock when vasopressin was incorporated into the treatment regimen.

A curveball in the VASST trial was the presence of corticosteroids in about 20% of patients in each group. In 2008, the evidence for administering corticosteroids in septic shock was not as compelling as today.[14,15] In a *post hoc* analysis, patients receiving vasopressin and corticosteroids had a lower 28-day mortality than those receiving norepinephrine and corticosteroids (35.9% vs. 44.7%, p=0.03), yielding an NNT of 11.4.[16] Anything to give our patients an edge, right? This intriguing result suggested a potential synergistic impact between vasopressin and corticosteroids, opening avenues for further exploration in septic shock management. However, here comes the reality check.

While the VASST trial could not conclusively settle the debate on vasopressin's overall benefits in septic shock, its findings underscored the importance of considering patient subgroups and potential therapeutic combinations to enhance outcomes. Though nuanced in its findings, the VASST trial was a pioneering exploration of vasopressin's role, which laid the foundation for subsequent research in the field.

VANISH (The VAsopressin vs. Norepinephrine as Initial Therapy in Septic SHock)
As a critical care medicine fellow in 2016, I vividly remember the impact of the VANISH trial when it was published. The academic community buzzed with discussion and anticipation. In contrast to its predecessor, the VASST trial, the authors of the VANISH trial embarked on a unique journey by incorporating the assessment of corticosteroid use into their study.[17] This change in approach led to a factorial 2 x 2 trial, pitting vasopressin against norepinephrine while also factoring in corticosteroid administration simultaneously. The VANISH trial allowed vasopressin to be titrated up to 0.06 U/min, marking an adjustment in the dosing strategy. It is worth noting that the VANISH trial enrolled fewer patients (n=409) than the VASST trial (n=778).

Spoiler Alert: The benefits observed in the VASST trial were not observed in the VANISH trial.[17] Like VASST, the VANISH trial did not demonstrate any statistically significant differences in 28-day mortality between the vasopressin and norepinephrine groups. However, it uncovered a noteworthy deviation from VASST: a reduction in the use of renal replacement therapy within the vasopressin group (25.4% vs. 35.3% [95% CI, −19.3% to −0.6%]). The considerable width of the confidence interval calls for statistical caution, but it implies an NNT of 10.1 to prevent one patient from requiring dialysis. This revelation offered a potential renal advantage for vasopressin use, an aspect not observed previously. Unlike VASST, the VANISH trial did not note the possible synergistic effect between corticosteroids and vasopressin. The interplay observed in the earlier trial, where vasopressin appeared to augment the benefits of corticosteroids, did not manifest here. These outcomes prompted the scientific community to delve deeper into the multifaceted relationship between vasopressin and corticosteroids and their effects on septic shock outcomes.

In their 2021 guidelines, the *Surviving Sepsis Campaign* acknowledged that "*some evidence suggests that vasopressin might be superior to norepinephrine in terms of clinical outcomes.*"[18]

Could cancer patients with septic shock benefit from first-line vasopressin?
VANCS II (VAsopressin versus Norepinephrine for the Management of Septic Shock in Cancer PatientS)
Medicine is not '*one-size-fits-all*'. Such recognition led to a pivotal RCT in 2019—known as VANCS II—exploring the role of vasopressin as a first-line agent in cancer patients with septic shock.[19] The rationale behind this exploration was multifaceted. For instance, a prominent consideration was the potential immunomodulatory effect of vasopressin. This thought process emerged from insights during two small animal studies where, to generalize, changes were observed in TNF-α and IL-6, among others.[22] While cautious about extrapolating findings from animal studies to humans, the potential effect on patient care justified further exploration.

Previous research offered hints about vasopressin's immunomodulatory effects.[6] For example, drawing from the VASST trial data involving 778 patients, researchers quantified cytokine levels in 394 patients.[60] Remarkably, patients treated with vasopressin exhibited a significant reduction in cytokine concentrations compared to those provided with norepinephrine at the 24-hour mark. However, it is worth noting that the VANISH trial did not replicate these benefits.[17] An essential context to remember is that norepinephrine was also recognized for its immunomodulatory impact during this period, emphasizing the complexity of the choices available.[22]

The VANCS II trial employed a titratable vasopressin strategy within the 0.01 to 0.06 U/min range rather than a fixed dose.[19] Interestingly, it also utilized a dosage range of 10-60 µg/min of norepinephrine. At some institutions, a 30 µg/min cap for norepinephrine exists. This practice is worth discussing; potential adjustment is explored in the *Norepinephrine* chapter. Unfortunately, this study involving 250 cancer patients found no significant differences when comparing vasopressin to norepinephrine.

What about vasopressin over norepinephrine for cardiac surgery-related vasoplegia?
VANCS: VAsopressin versus Norepinephrine in Patients with Vasoplegia Shock after Cardiac Surgery
For those unfamiliar with cardiac surgery-related vasoplegia—a type of distributive shock—please refer to *The Basics* chapter for a more detailed

explanation. In the VANCS trial, 300 patients were enrolled in an RCT evaluating the efficacy of norepinephrine compared with vasopressin in cardiac surgery-related vasoplegia.[8]

The primary outcome measure focused on a composite endpoint incorporating mortality and severe complications. Notably, severe complications included incidents such as stroke, mechanical ventilation for over 48 hours, sternal wound infection, reoperation, and acute renal failure. Vasopressin demonstrated an advantage in this primary outcome, achieved only 32% of the time in the vasopressin group compared to 49% in the norepinephrine group. This translated into an NNT of 5.9. Particularly noteworthy was the marked reduction in the incidence of acute renal failure in the vasopressin group (10.3%) compared to the norepinephrine group (35.8%), further underscoring the benefits of vasopressin with a remarkably low NNT of 3.9. This renal advantage also resonated with findings from the VANISH trial, which demonstrated promising renal outcomes.[17] Additionally, using vasopressin significantly reduced the length of stay in the ICU and the hospital, reflecting shorter recovery times than norepinephrine.

Exploring secondary outcomes, including adverse events, the incidence of atrial fibrillation—typically associated with norepinephrine—was markedly lower in the vasopressin group (63.8%) compared to the norepinephrine group (82.1%), with an associated NNT of 5.5. It is worth noting that these atrial fibrillation rates may appear higher than some clinicians typically encounter. Nevertheless, no significant differences were observed in other adverse events, such as digital ischemia, mesenteric ischemia, hyponatremia, or myocardial infarction, signifying vasopressin as a preferable choice from a safety perspective.

An interesting aside is the authors' measurement of plasma vasopressin levels in the VANCS trial. Patients who had undergone cardiopulmonary bypass surgery exhibited lower plasma vasopressin levels compared to those with septic shock. This disparity was attributed to reduced vasopressin production and its release into circulation among cardiac surgery patients. This intriguing insight sheds light on the complex dynamics of vasopressin regulation in distinct clinical contexts.[8] The findings from the VANCS trial align with the results of a prior, albeit smaller, study involving 40 patients who received vasopressin following cardiac surgery.[7] In this earlier study, which focused on improving MAP and reducing the requirement for vasopressors, vasopressin demonstrated its potential to enhance hemodynamic stability.

Should we prophylactically administer vasopressin to patients at risk for cardiac surgery-related vasoplegia?
In 2003, this question was explored by Morales *et al.* based on established evidence identifying ACE inhibitors as a significant risk factor for cardiac surgery-related vasoplegia.[20] The study—involving 27 patients—randomized subjects to receive either vasopressin at 0.03 U/min or a placebo 20 minutes before surgery.

Both groups received standard post-procedure medical management, regardless of whether they received vasopressin or a placebo. The outcomes favored the vasopressin group, demonstrating more effective catecholamine-sparing effects, reduced hypotension episodes, and a shorter ICU stay. This approach may not be prevalent in clinical practice but holds merit in cases where the risk factors align.

Given the findings of these landmark trials, can vasopressin be a first-line agent?
Evaluating the collective evidence from landmark trials, including VASST, VANISH, and VANCS II, it is clear that vasopressin is non-inferior to norepinephrine.[6,17,19] While it may not be a superior option, it is viable for specific patient subgroups. One such example is patients with atrial fibrillation with a rapid ventricular rate, a topic we will delve into later.

Per the *Surviving Sepsis Campaign* guidelines, the primary factor precluding vasopressin from the status of a first-line agent is the higher cost and lower availability compared to norepinephrine.[18] However, these considerations have evolved since the 2021 guideline update, with a subsequent decrease in vasopressin's cost projected to increase availability. However, the evidence does not yet substantiate vasopressin as a replacement for norepinephrine in the hierarchy of vasopressors for septic shock. Nonetheless, vasopressin emerges as a potential first-line candidate for cardiac surgery-related vasoplegia patients.[8]

When should we add vasopressin as a second-line agent in septic shock?
Determining the optimal point at which to introduce vasopressin as a second-line agent in the management of septic shock is a challenge. The 2021 *Surviving Sepsis Campaign* suggests considering vasopressin when norepinephrine reaches a dosage of 0.25-0.5 µg/kg/min.[18] Nevertheless, even these authors acknowledge the variability in the threshold for initiating vasopressin among various studies. The VASST trial offers some guidance, revealing improved survival rates for patients requiring less than 15 µg/min of norepinephrine when initiating vasopressin.[6]

Traditionally, some clinicians have considered vasopressin initiation when norepinephrine dosages reach double digits in µg/min, often aided by hemodynamic monitoring to distinguish distributive shock from cardiogenic elements. However, the lack of definitive answers persists due to the absence of well-designed studies on this topic. Clinicians have had to rely on *post-hoc* analyses to hypothesize when to introduce the second agent based on time and norepinephrine-equivalent considerations.[21] A retrospective study involving 1610 patients highlighted that waiting longer to initiate vasopressin correlated with worse outcomes.[23] The study found that lower norepinephrine-equivalent doses and lower lactate levels at vasopressin initiation led to improved prognoses.

Additionally, for every 10 μg/min increase in norepinephrine-equivalent vasopressor dosage, in-hospital mortality increased by 20.7%.

A retrospective study including 385 patients who received vasopressin within seven hours of admission demonstrated improved outcomes compared to those in whom vasopressin administration was delayed.[35] Remarkably, the early vasopressin group experienced fewer incidents of acute kidney injury (AKI) and fewer initiations of renal replacement therapy. In addition, these patients demonstrated shorter durations of mechanical ventilation, reduced lengths of stay in the ICU, and lower all-cause in-hospital mortality rates. Earlier may be better.

Will we ever get a dedicated study on vasopressin to see if there is a mortality benefit over other vasopressors?
Dedicated research exploring whether vasopressin exhibits a mortality benefit over other vasopressors remains elusive under current clinical trial paradigms. Paul Young—a respected figure in critical care research—estimates that a study adequately powered to establish mortality effects would necessitate an approximately 44,000-patient cohort with septic shock.[24] However, the myriad challenges inherent to such a massive trial have thus far deterred such an undertaking.

Is vasopressin more gentle on the pulmonary vasculature than norepinephrine?
During my training, I was educated that vasopressin is superior to norepinephrine in patients with pulmonary hypertension or right heart failure after cardiac surgery due to the minimal or lack of effect on the pulmonary vasculature. The relevance of this information, especially given the potential clinical implications, prompted an in-depth exploration into its origins and validity. It is imperative to realize that the wrong vasopressor in this patient population could cause serious harm.

Early canine studies investigated vasopressin's effects on the pulmonary artery, revealing reduced pulmonary resistance and pulmonary artery pressure (PAP) during vasopressin administration.[25,26] However, a 2007 retrospective study—primarily involving patients with septic and cardiac surgery-related vasoplegia—raised many questions.[27] This study compared two vasopressin doses—0.033 U/hr and 0.067 U/hr—to norepinephrine. Remarkably, patients receiving the higher vasopressin dose (0.067 U/hr) displayed lower mean PAP compared to those receiving the lower dose (0.033 U/hr). The authors contemplated whether this outcome stemmed from the higher vasopressin doses leading to reduced norepinephrine requirements.

In 2014, subsequent research featured an *in vitro* analysis of vasopressin, norepinephrine, phenylephrine, and metaraminol on human tissue rings from both radial and pulmonary arteries.[28] The study's comprehensive examination was enabled by obtaining tissue from patients undergoing coronary artery bypass grafting (CABG) and lung resection procedures. The study affirmed vasopressin's robust impact on radial arteries, with a minimal effect on the pulmonary arteries. Notably, while the study focused on the primary pulmonary artery, it remained unclear how vasopressin affected the smaller pulmonary arteries, which play a more significant role in pulmonary vascular resistance (PVR).

Given this evidence, one can reasonably infer that vasopressin tends to be gentler on the pulmonary vasculature than norepinephrine. Consequently, vasopressin represents a favorable choice when managing patients with elevated pulmonary artery pressures, particularly in cases where clinical circumstances warrant such consideration.

Would vasopressin be gentle on the pulmonary artery pressures after cardiac surgery with pulmonary hypertension?

Beginning in 2007, a series of smaller studies in the cardiac surgery patient population emerged, collectively demonstrating that vasopressin effectively improved hemodynamics without exacerbating underlying pulmonary hypertension.[29] A study involving 50 patients requiring milrinone for right ventricular dysfunction following cardiac surgery compared vasopressin and norepinephrine.

The findings underscored the combination of milrinone and vasopressin as optimal for managing right heart failure, attributing this to an improved pulmonary vascular resistance to systemic vascular resistance (PVR/SVR) ratio.[30] In another 20-patient study, which randomized patients to receive either norepinephrine or vasopressin after cardiac surgery, no increases in PVR or PAP were noted in the vasopressin group, further affirming vasopressin as a favorable option for patients with pulmonary hypertension.[31]

Does vasopressin favorably affect the kidneys?

The compelling prospect of renal benefits associated with vasopressin use has been a recurring theme in various studies. The VASST and VANISH trials suggested that vasopressin may confer renal advantages in patients with septic shock.[6,17] A post hoc analysis of the VASST trial revealed that patients at risk of developing renal failure benefited from vasopressin therapy.[33] A meta-analysis pooling data from RCTs within this patient population further supported the idea, reporting a diminished requirement for renal replacement therapy when patients received vasopressin.[34]

Does vasopressin retain efficacy in acidosis?

There is a prevailing belief in our community that vasopressin maintains effectiveness in acidotic conditions better than other vasopressors due to the resilience of V1a receptors to acidemia, unlike α-1 receptors. Early research— such as a 1992 rat tail artery study—supports this, demonstrating vasopressin's preserved response in metabolic acidosis. This finding is often cited as evidence of its robust action in acidotic states.[36-38] However, real-world data are limited.

One study demonstrated higher rates of ROSC with vasopressin in cardiac arrest patients with pH < 7.2.[39] A more recent retrospective study published in 2022 involving 1350 patients contradicts this, indicating vasopressin's efficacy is also compromised in acidemia.[40] The data are not conclusive enough to firmly answer this question, especially since patients with severe acidosis often require multiple vasopressors. For strategies on correcting acidosis to potentiate vasopressor efficacy, the BICAR-ICU trial offers valuable insights.[41]

What adverse effects are associated with vasopressin?
Like all medications discussed in this text, vasopressin carries the potential for adverse effects. In critically ill patients, there is an inherent risk of complications such as mesenteric ischemia, acute coronary syndrome, and digit ischemia. Notably, two systematic reviews with meta-analyses indicate that the incidence of digit ischemia may be higher with vasopressin than other vasopressors.[34,44] In contrast, vasopressin may pose a lower risk of arrhythmias than norepinephrine.

A retrospective study by Ferenchick et al. highlighted an intriguing potential side effect: the development of diabetes insipidus (DI) following the cessation of vasopressin infusion, with a reported occurrence rate of 1.53%.[45] While the precise mechanism remains speculative, the authors suggest that DI could result from the downregulation of V2 receptors due to supraphysiological doses of vasopressin. I have yet to encounter this condition in my practice, which suggests it may require a more vigilant approach to detect.

What is the dosing range for vasopressin for shock?
The Surviving Sepsis Campaign endorses a standardized dose of 0.03 U/min for vasopressin in the management of septic shock.[18] However, this is not the only dosing regimen that is safe and effective in clinical practice. Several studies indicate that vasopressin dosing is flexible:
• Dünser MW et al. have utilized a dose of 0.067 U/min.[13]
• Similarly, Luckner G et al. reported using 0.067 U/min.[27]
• The VASST trial included a range from 0.01 to 0.03 U/min.[6]
• The VANISH trial explored doses up to 0.06 U/min.[17]
These variations highlight that while there is a recommended dose, clinical judgment and individual patient needs can guide dosing within an established safe range.

0.03 U/min or 0.04 U/min for septic shock?
This appears to be largely dependent on institutional preferences. I have encountered hospitals that use either dosage. I have observed variations even within different units of the same institution. The Surviving Sepsis Campaign

recommends a standard dosing of 0.03 U/min.[18] However, does this recommendation align with the evidence?

Conducting a prospective study comparing these two dosages would take considerable work. Fortunately, we can refer to a retrospective analysis of 1536 patients that sheds light on this debate.[51] This study evaluated whether a dosage of 0.04 U/min resulted in a more favorable hemodynamic response than 0.03 U/min, specifically looking at improvements in MAP and catecholamine requirements. The findings? There was no significant difference between the two dosages. Choosing 0.03 U/min aligns with standard recommendations and offers a 25% increase in product per bag—essentially 'more for free.' Thus, this approach could also lead to cost savings, potentially contributing to hospital funds for employee raises.

Is it possible to exceed the standard dosing of 0.03 U/min for vasopressin?
I honestly do not see why not. In dire circumstances where a patient's life hangs in the balance, going beyond the guideline-recommended dosage may become necessary. The decision to do so should always be grounded in a cautious risk-versus-benefit assessment. Patient consent, or at least informed agreement, becomes even more relevant when considering doses that surpass established guidelines. The objective is clear: to save lives when all other options have been exhausted.

Is vasopressin titratable?
The question of whether vasopressin is titratable is one that frequently arises in clinical practice. While guidelines often provide specific dosing recommendations, numerous clinical trials have successfully employed titratable doses of vasopressin without encountering adverse effects.[6,8,17,19] This suggests there's room for flexibility in vasopressin dosing, allowing for customization based on individual patient needs. Adjusting the dose based on the clinical context while assessing the risk-benefit ratio remains prudent.

What is the highest published dose of vasopressin in the medical literature?
A 2007 cardiac surgery-based study pushed the conventional limits of vasopressin dosing. Nine patients were initiated at 0.05 U/min and gradually escalated to 0.1 U/min, pushing the boundaries of conventional vasopressin dosing.[29] Before this study, the highest dose observed was 0.067 U/min.[13,27] Although these patients remained on these high doses for an average of 4.0 ± 2.3 days due to refractory vasoplegia, they did not experience adverse effects attributed to vasopressin.[29] In another instance, a more daring attempt was made, utilizing up to 0.2 U/min of vasopressin in a 23-patient trial.[52] No adverse events were noted there.

According to the *Vasostrict* package insert, the maximum recommended dose for post-cardiotomy shock is 0.1 U/min.[2] In the case of septic shock, it is 0.07 U/min.

This underscores the importance of flexibility in vasopressin dosing, as patients' specific needs can vary significantly. Rigid adherence to a one-size-fits-all approach may not be the most appropriate course of action in certain critical scenarios.

Which should we wean off first: vasopressin or norepinephrine?
Determining the order in which to wean vasopressin and norepinephrine can be an essential decision for septic shock management. In 2019, a systematic review and meta-analysis, including six studies and 957 patients, attempted to determine if norepinephrine or vasopressin should be weaned off first in septic shock patients.[53] In this work, four of the six studies illustrated a clear benefit with lower incidences of hypotension when norepinephrine was discontinued before vasopressin.

None of the studies suggest that vasopressin should be stopped first. It is speculated that vasopressin's longer half-life and the persistence of its deficiency contribute to these findings. In 2020, another systematic review and meta-analysis was able to dig up eight studies with 1164 patients and concluded the same.[54] It will not work every time, but weaning norepinephrine first is what we should do.

Should vasopressin be weaned or abruptly discontinued?
When patients turn the corner, the choice between abrupt discontinuation and tapering of vasopressin becomes prominent. A retrospective study of 958 septic shock patients concluded that abrupt discontinuation was associated with a shorter vasopressin duration.[55] In addition, vasopressin had to be restarted fewer times in the abrupt discontinuation group than in the tapered discontinuation group (5.7% vs. 11.7%, p <0.001). The primary outcome was time to ICU discharge, with no difference between the two groups. Hit the off button on the pump and discontinue it abruptly. Keep in mind that medicine is not '*one size fits all*.' Flexibility in clinical decision-making is essential, as each patient may respond differently to vasopressin discontinuation.

Does vasopressin produce the same immunoparalysis that norepinephrine and other catecholamines do?
Unfortunately, human studies investigating whether vasopressin—like norepinephrine and other catecholamines—induces immunoparalysis have been elusive due to most patients on vasopressin being concurrently administered norepinephrine. As a result, it becomes challenging to tease out the direct effects of vasopressin.[22]

Animal studies have offered intriguing insights, suggesting anti-inflammatory properties, including less TNF-α, IL-6, and IL-10 production than norepinephrine in porcine sepsis models. Studies in mice with sepsis have also hinted at local anti-inflammatory effects in the lung.[32] The unanswered question regarding whether vasopressin elicits immunoparalysis highlights a significant knowledge gap.

Is vasopressin utilized for GI bleeds?
I have heard the commentary of gastrointestinal (GI) bleed-dose of vasopressin but have never reached for it. Regardless, it does have its place in the guidelines for managing *Portal Hypertensive Bleeding in Cirrhosis*, specifically for acute variceal hemorrhage.[42] Here, the splanchnic vasoconstrictive effects of vasopressin, typically undesirable, become beneficial. While sepsis management calls for doses around 0.03 U/min, vasopressin dosing for variceal bleeding is more aggressive, beginning with a continuous infusion of 0.2-0.4 U/min and potentially escalating to 0.8 U/min.

Co-administration with nitroglycerin as a wingman is advised to mitigate vasopressin's adverse effects. However, it is worth noting that these dosing strategies, trialed in 1990, were less effective than using a Sengstaken-Blakemore tube for esophageal varices or a Linton-Nachlas tube for gastric varices.[43] Thus, vasopressin for GI bleeds is a secondary or last-ditch option when other treatments are exhausted or unavailable.

Should vasopressin be utilized in cardiac arrest?
Researching patients who have suffered a cardiac arrest poses formidable challenges. Considerations include the logistics of patient enrollment, randomization, the arrest setting (in-hospital versus out-of-hospital)—the type of cardiac rhythm (shockable or non-shockable)—and whether the drug is utilized alone or in conjunction with others.

In the ACLS guidelines, vasopressin was listed until the 2015 update, when it was no longer recommended as the sole vasoactive drug during ACLS.[46] The rationale for using vasopressin in the first place was based on several studies: firstly, higher endogenous vasopressin levels were observed in cardiac arrest survivors compared to non-survivors; secondly, an RCT involving 40 patients, along with some case studies, suggested benefits of vasopressin over epinephrine.[47] However, a pivotal 336-patient trial comparing vasopressin to epinephrine demonstrated no advantage,[48] leading the American Heart Association to advise against vasopressin as an epinephrine alternative in cardiac arrest.[46]

Despite these findings, a total dismissal of vasopressin entirely may be premature. The same study that led to its removal demonstrated improved rates of return of spontaneous circulation (ROSC) with vasopressin in instances where bystander CPR was performed and the arrest was witnessed.[48] Although initial statistical analyses were promising, subsequent analyses questioned these findings.

More recently, a combination of vasopressin and methylprednisolone was associated with higher ROSC rates in an RCT of 512 patients with in-hospital cardiac arrests.[49] A subsequent systematic review and meta-analysis acknowledged significant limitations and recommended further large-scale studies. The review concluded that vasopressin and glucocorticoids together may improve ROSC rates compared to placebo.[50]

FUN FACTS!

Discovery of Vasopressin: Arginine vasopressin (AVP) was discovered by Oliver and Schäfer in 1895, who uncovered vasopressin's role in blood pressure regulation.[3,56] In 1955, Vincent du Vigneaud was awarded the Nobel Prize in Chemistry for isolating and synthesizing vasopressin (and oxytocin) and elucidating its antidiuretic and vasopressor properties.[3,57]

Why Does Vasopressin Have Multiple Names? The various terms for vasopressin, including arginine vasopressin (AVP) and anti-diuretic hormone (ADH), can be confusing. These different names reflect the hormone's diverse functions and the evolution of its nomenclature over time.

FDA Approval: 2014.[2]

Trade Names of Vasopressin: Vasostrict, Reverpleg, Empressin, Pressyn, Cpressin, Cevas-40, and Cpressin P.[58]

The Price Surge of Vasopressin (2014-2021): Between 2014 and 2021, vasopressin experienced a dramatic price increase, primarily due to the Unapproved Drugs Initiative by Congress, which granted exclusive manufacturing and selling rights to a single company.[59] This exclusivity led to a staggering price hike of 5,400%. The good news is that this exclusivity ended in September 2021, allowing for market competition and potentially more affordable pricing.

Citations

eddyjoemd.com/vasopressin-citations

06: TERLIPRESSIN

I envisioned terlipressin as a vasopressor that would transform the scope of management in shock patients as it is a more targeted form of vasopressin. However, unfortunately, things did not work out that way. It is like having a renaissance of sorts after being FDA-approved for hepatorenal syndrome in 2022.[3]

What is the mechanism of action of terlipressin?
Terlipressin, a synthetic vasopressin analog, differs notably in its affinity for vasopressin receptors. Specifically, terlipressin has a higher affinity for the V1a receptor than vasopressin.[1,2] This higher affinity implies terlipressin has a reduced impact on the V2 receptor, which is associated with antidiuretic effects. According to the package insert, terlipressin exhibits twice the selectivity for V1 receptors over V2 receptors.[3] This receptor selectivity suggests terlipressin should have less of an "anti-diuretic" impact than vasopressin. The reduced action on V2 receptors is advantageous, as it potentially leads to fewer antidiuretic effects and a diminished prothrombotic impact, often mediated through *Von Willebrand* factor release.[4] Terlipressin is a prodrug, which is converted to lysine-vasopressin (not arginine-vasopressin) via endothelial peptidases to exert vasopressor effects.[5]

Considering the MAP = CO x SVR equation, terlipressin increases systemic vascular resistance (SVR) in order to improve the mean arterial pressure (MAP). There is no direct effect on the cardiac output (CO).

What is the half-life of terlipressin?
The half-life of terlipressin is approximately six hours.[3] This relatively extended half-life allows for its administration in intermittent boluses rather than necessitating a continuous infusion.[6] This mode of administration can be particularly advantageous in clinical settings where IV access is limited. Such situations might include cases with multiple incompatible infusions running concurrently, a shortage of infusion pumps, or nursing staff limitations.

Did terlipressin ever have a chance to shine in septic shock?
Terlipressin's role in septic shock has been a subject of research, but its efficacy and safety remain debated. Early smaller studies suggested terlipressin, akin to vasopressin, could reduce norepinephrine requirements in septic shock patients.[7,8] These initial findings, while intriguing, were limited in scope, emphasizing the need for larger, more comprehensive randomized controlled trials (RCTs).

In 2018, a notable RCT involving 617 patients with septic shock was conducted to evaluate terlipressin.[9] Participants were administered either terlipressin or norepinephrine as the primary vasopressor. Spoiler alert: the trial was stopped early for futility at 50% enrollment. The primary outcome was mortality, for which there was no difference. The results demonstrated no significant difference in mortality or secondary outcomes like SOFA scores and vasopressor-free days post-randomization.

A key concern raised by this trial was the high incidence of adverse effects, mainly digital ischemia, which occurred in 12.6% of patients receiving terlipressin. Take a second to process that. More than 1 in 10 patients will have digital ischemia. This rate of ischemia surpasses what is typically observed with vasopressin. Critics have posited that the terlipressin dosages might have been higher than optimal.[10] The trial also noted a higher frequency of diarrhea in the terlipressin group (2.72% vs. 0.35%).

Current research does not indicate further standalone terlipressin studies are planned, as per clinicaltrials.gov. The *Surviving Sepsis Campaign* Guidelines have since issued a weak recommendation against using terlipressin in septic shock.[11] Echoing Mårtensson and Gordon's perspective, terlipressin may be unnecessary in sepsis if vasopressin, a less adverse-effect-prone alternative, is available.[4]

The utility of terlipressin in septic shock has also been assessed in two systematic reviews and meta-analyses.[12,13] Zhu et al.'s review, involving 928 patients, found no mortality benefits but indicated a possible reduction in mechanical ventilation duration.[12] Conversely, Huang et al.'s analysis of 850 patients suggested a mortality reduction in those under 60 and potential renal function improvements, albeit with a higher risk of digital ischemia.[13] However, the most extensive study in these reviews, involving 617 patients by Liu et al., significantly influences these findings. Compared to the next largest study with only 84 patients, the potential benefits observed are overshadowed by alternatives like norepinephrine's established efficacy and safety profile.

Is terlipressin better as an adjunct vasopressor in septic shock?
The potential of terlipressin as an adjunct to norepinephrine in septic shock has garnered interest, especially considering the established use of vasopressin in similar roles.[14] A 50-patient RCT investigated the efficacy of combining norepinephrine with terlipressin compared to norepinephrine alone.[10] The results of this study were notable. The group receiving both norepinephrine and terlipressin demonstrated a quicker reduction in SOFA scores at the 12-hour mark and experienced a shorter duration on vasopressors among survivors. These findings suggest a potential benefit of using terlipressin as an adjunct therapy.

However, a significant concern arose from this study: the incidence of digital ischemia. Alarmingly, 28% (7 out of 25) of patients in the combination therapy group developed digital ischemia, even though terlipressin was administered for only 12 hours. This recurrence of digital ischemia across various studies signals a considerable risk associated with terlipressin use. Let's stick to using vasopressin.

Terlipressin vs. vasopressin: who would win?
Terlipressin's reduced impact on V2 receptors, theoretically leading to lesser fluid retention, diminished thrombocytopenia, and improved CO, might suggest it as the preferable option.[15] These attributes hint at potentially superior patient outcomes with terlipressin. Evidence from a 45-patient study indicated no significant difference in overall outcomes between terlipressin and vasopressin.[8]

This finding suggests that the presumed advantages of terlipressin may not translate into markedly improved clinical results. It is crucial to note that such a study's limited size may not effectively capture the subtle differences between the two vasopressors. A more extensive, well-powered study is necessary to draw more definitive conclusions. The lack of substantial data favoring terlipressin means that availability and clinical familiarity should guide the choice between it and vasopressin.

Could terlipressin improve renal perfusion in septic shock?
The potential of terlipressin to enhance renal perfusion in septic shock remains an area of interest despite the absence of such findings in the extensive RCT by Liu et al.[9] A 2022 pilot study involving 22 patients, where terlipressin was added to norepinephrine for treating septic shock, has sparked further curiosity into this possibility.[16] This study reported improvements in renal perfusion and increased stroke volume, presenting intriguing yet preliminary insights. However, it is essential to approach these findings with caution, considering the limited scale and scope of the pilot study.

Like vasopressin, can terlipressin relax the pulmonary vasculature?
Investigating porcine models can offer valuable insights for future human research. In a notable *in vivo* study, pigs subjected to pulmonary emboli were administered terlipressin.[17] The outcomes for the terlipressin group, when compared with control subjects, revealed a decrease in pulmonary artery pressure and an elevation in SVR. However, the observed reduction in pulmonary vascular resistance did not reach statistical significance. A direct comparison between terlipressin and vasopressin focusing on their pulmonary vascular effects could reshape clinical approaches, especially in managing complex pulmonary embolism cases. Such a trial could provide critical data to inform and refine treatment protocols in this challenging patient demographic.

Is terlipressin an option for cardiac surgery-related vasoplegia?
A 2019 review article on cardiac surgery-related vasoplegia by Levy et al. suggests a potential use of terlipressin for this patient population due to its

mechanism of action.[18] Unfortunately, there are no published or ongoing studies of terlipressin for this patient population. We should stay away for now.

What adverse effects should we watch out for?
Digital ischemia is the number one adverse effect on the list, as observed in various trials and meta-analyses.[9,15] Diarrhea is number two (insert winking emoji here).[9]

Why is terlipressin indicated for type 1 hepatorenal syndrome?
Terlipressin's indication for Type 1 Hepatorenal Syndrome (HRS) is rooted in its unique renal and portal hemodynamics effects. HRS, particularly its Type 1 variant, presents a grim prognosis with rapid deterioration of renal function, distinguishing it from the more gradual Type 2 HRS.[19] For context, terlipressin, often utilized alongside albumin, has been a focus of treatment trials for HRS since 2001.[20] It offers an alternative to traditional therapies like octreotide, albumin, norepinephrine, midodrine, and dopamine, aimed at reversing HRS. Terlipressin is favored due to its ability to reduce portal hypertension and increase renal blood flow by improving the MAP and effective arterial volume.[3]

A 2018 systematic review and meta-analysis revealed that terlipressin led to HRS reversal in 42% of patients, compared to 26.2% in control groups, highlighting its potential in HRS management.[20] However, its superiority over norepinephrine in reversing Type 1 HRS and improving renal outcomes needed to be established. Despite this, the European Association for the Study of the Liver (EASL) endorses terlipressin and albumin as the primary treatment for acute kidney injury in HRS.[21]

The CONFIRM study, a Phase III trial, further assessed the efficacy and safety of terlipressin plus albumin in Type 1 HRS patients.[22] This pivotal trial, involving 300 participants, compared terlipressin plus albumin against placebo. You read that correctly: placebo. Not norepinephrine, which previous data found to be equivalent in reversing Type 1 HRS to terlipressin.[20] Its primary endpoint was the confirmed reversal of HRS, achieving a 32% success rate with terlipressin versus 17% with placebo. The study illuminated various secondary benefits of terlipressin, such as sustained HRS reversal without renal replacement therapy and effectiveness in patients with Systemic Inflammatory Response Syndrome (SIRS).

In 2022, the FDA approved terlipressin for use in the United States, albeit with notable caution for patients with respiratory failure.[3] The black box warning advises against initiating terlipressin in patients with oxygen saturations below 90% and recommends discontinuation if oxygen saturation falls below this threshold during treatment. This caution stems from the 22 respiratory-related deaths observed in the CONFIRM study within 90 days.

FUN FACTS!

Alternative Names: Terlivaz, and scientifically as triacyl-lysine vasopressin.

FDA Approval Date: September 12, 2022.

Citations

eddyjoemd.com/terlipressin-citations

07: SELEPRESSIN

Have you ever heard of Selepressin? It wouldn't be surprising if you had not. In 2016, as a critical care medicine fellow, I attended my first Society of Critical Care Medicine (SCCM) conference in Orlando, FL. I enthusiastically participated with my co-fellow and close friend Casey Bryant in a session titled *"Bench-Pressing in the ICU: Which Vasopressor Agent Should I Choose for My Patient?"* During this session, Dr. Lakhmir S. Chawla introduced selepressin as a novel vasopressor in the pipeline. It was exciting news, and we anticipated seeing it in our ICUs in the near future. However, what happened next?

What is the mechanism of action of selepressin?
Selepressin—a synthetic vasopressin analog—is a selective V1a receptor agonist.[7] In contrast, vasopressin activates the V1b and V2 receptors in addition to the V1a receptors. Selepressin aimed to avoid unnecessary receptor stimulation.

The net effect of selepressin on the MAP = CO x SVR equation is, like vasopressin, an increase in systemic vascular resistance (SVR). No direct impact is noted on the cardiac output (CO).

Why did we initiate human trials with selepressin?
Let's briefly review the timeline of fundamental studies that led to human trials:
- 2011: Superior to vasopressin and norepinephrine in ovine (sheep) fecal peritonitis-induced septic shock.[2]
- 2012: Attenuated vascular dysfunction and fluid accumulation in ovine severe sepsis.[3]
- 2014: Outperformed vasopressin in blocking vascular leak in ovine pseudomonas pneumonia sepsis.[4]
- 2016: Demonstrated superiority to vasopressin and norepinephrine in maintaining MAP and CI while reducing lung edema and cumulative fluid balance in ovine septic shock due to fecal peritonitis.[5]
- 2020: Demonstrated protective effects against endothelial barrier dysfunction in bench research.[6]
- 2020: Equivalent risk for mesenteric ischemia as vasopressin[7]

What human studies made us optimistic?
In the Phase I trial, selepressin was infused into healthy volunteers without causing any issues. Although these study findings were not formally published, they were referenced in another article.[8] It should be noted that Phase I trials primarily aim to evaluate the safety of the therapeutic on humans. Following the success of this trial, it was determined that Selepressin was safe to proceed to Phase IIa—*i.e.,* efficacy study through these trials.

In the Phase IIa trial, selepressin's efficacy was investigated in 53 patients with early septic shock.[8] Early septic shock was defined as hypotension lasting over 2 hours with norepinephrine being administered. Patients were randomized to receive selepressin at one of three doses to maintain a MAP $\geq$ 65 mmHg, while the control group received a *placebo*. Patients received open-label norepinephrine as needed to achieve the MAP goal. The trial's primary outcomes included stabilizing MAP (>60 mmHg) without open-label norepinephrine at various assessment points and cumulative doses. Secondary endpoints encompassed selepressin's pharmacodynamics/pharmacokinetic profile, adverse effects, cumulative fluid balance, and morbidity. As a result, the optimal dose was determined to be 2.5 ng/kg/min.

Enthusiasm spread across the critical care community when these results were published. Several benefits were observed, including sparing norepinephrine usage in septic shock, enabling faster weaning, improving net fluid balance, and reducing time on mechanical ventilation.

When did selepressin receive its reality check?
The Selepressin Evaluation Programme for Sepsis-Induced Shock—Adaptive Clinical Trial (SEPSIS-ACT) was a Phase IIb/III trial published in 2019.[9] This trial had two phases, akin to '*Avengers: Infinity War*' and '*Avengers: Endgame*,' but with a less satisfying conclusion. Spoiler alert: The trial was terminated early due to futility.

This 817-patient randomized controlled trial (RCT) reevaluated the three dosing strategies from the Phase IIa trial but then confirmed the efficacy of the optimal dosing regimen in septic shock. Unfortunately, the composite endpoint of vasopressor-free and ventilator-free days was not met. As a result, the previously observed benefits of norepinephrine weaning and reduction in the time on mechanical ventilation were absent. Several secondary outcomes were also negative. Adverse event rates were similar in both groups.

Despite this negative trial, some positives can be gleaned from the data. Like vasopressin, selepressin did have a norepinephrine-sparing effect. Results demonstrated that patients exhibited less cardiovascular dysfunction, higher urine output, and a lower net fluid balance within the first 24 hours—however more benefits than these were needed to secure FDA approval.

Is cardiac surgery-related vasoplegia a possible indication?
Considering the vasopressin benefits demonstrated in patients with cardiac surgery-related vasoplegia in the VANCS trial, it is worth wondering if selepressin could be beneficial in this clinical scenario.[13] Selepressin offers potential advantages, such as blocking microvascular leaks, not contributing to fluid accumulation, and not promoting microvascular thrombosis related to von Willebrand factor release.[10,11] The question arises of whether Ferring

Pharmaceuticals will consider revisiting selepressin for trials in this patient population.

Any potential anti-inflammatory effects?
Yes, selepressin has anti-inflammatory effects, possibly due to its ability to reduce the production of pro-inflammatory cytokines.[12] What does this mean clinically? We may never find out.

FUN FACTS!
Origin Story: In 2010, selepressin was launched as FE 202158. I found several other names in the literature, including cysteine-phenylalanine-isoleucine-homoglutamine-asparagine-cysteine-proline-ornithine(isopropyl)-glycine-NH2[1] and Phe2-Orn8-Vasotocin (POV)[2].

Citations
eddyjoemd.com/selepressin-citations

08: DOPAMINE

Dopamine's story is a rollercoaster. Once the first choice for vasopressors, it is now more likely to gather dust in the pharmacy basement or be pulled out of the drug dispensing machine as it has expired. During my residency, I recall dopamine being stored in the crash carts so we could promptly hang a pre-mixed vasopressor during a code. Multiple clinical trials demonstrated no benefit, even within the decompensated heart failure population.[1,2] Nonetheless, dopamine is still prescribed in certain situations, right?

What is the mechanism of action of dopamine?
Dopamine is an endogenous catecholamine and the precursor of norepinephrine. It acts on four dose-dependent receptors (see next section), including dopaminergic receptor Types 1 and 2, α-1 and β-1 adrenergic receptors. In some studies, dopaminergic receptor Type 4 is also considered in the mechanism of action.[3]

Dopamine's dose-dependent effects make the result of our MAP = CO X SVR equation tricky. Patients could experience decreases or increases in their mean arterial pressure (MAP). This is due to variable effects on systemic vascular resistance (SVR). Increases in cardiac output (CO) are seen with the intermediate doses.

What is the deal with these dose-dependent effects?
Dopamine is reported to be dose-dependent, but it is also clinical-scenario-dependent. I was always skeptical of how the delineations were so transparent as to what was low, intermediate, and high dosing. However, my skepticism was further exacerbated when these delineations varied depending on the article studied. To assign authority, we will utilize the package insert (PI) as the guide.[4]

0.5-2 µg/kg/min: Dopamine causes vasodilation through dopaminergic receptors at these low infusion rates. Consequently, it is reported that dopamine increases urine output due to increased glomerular filtration rate, renal blood flow, and sodium excretion. However, due to the vasodilation at these doses, hypotension could occur.[4] At these 'low' doses, dopamine could result in a decrease in SVR.

2-10 µg/kg/min: These intermediate rates of dopamine stimulate the β-1 adrenergic receptors, which lead to increased contractility and chronotropy (*i.e.*, an increase in heart rate). Note that these doses still have limited or zero impact on the α receptors.[4] Thus, we observe the possible cardiac benefits of dopamine as it improves patients' stroke volume (SV) (due to the contractility component) and heart rate (HR). At these 'intermediate' doses, dopamine could increase CO.

10-20 µg/kg/min: Higher dopamine doses result primarily in vasoconstriction. The α-1 adrenergic receptor activity predominates, which enhances the SVR and, therefore, increases the MAP.[4]

Other sources cite the same effects on the low, intermediate, and higher infusion thresholds but with varying doses. However, this is where things may get perplexing. Some data claim low dose as < 5 µg/kg/min, intermediate as 5-10 µg/kg/min, and high as 10-20 µg/kg/min.[5,6] Similarly, other research works reveal low as 0.5-3 µg/kg/min, intermediate as 3-10 µg/kg/min, and high as 10-20 µg/kg/min.[7] Another research article defines intermediate as 5-15 µg/kg/min.[8] Which of these studies is the most accurate? Does it even matter?

Are these dose-dependent effects real?
It would be nice if titrating dopamine to a particular dose accomplishes the required results, but it does not.[3] Patients in shock do not follow the same rules as those with normal physiological conditions.[10] The infusion rate cannot predict dopamine plasma levels.[3] Moreover, one cannot claim a dose-dependent effect if we do not know the plasma level in a patient.

Adding salt to the wound, there is an overlap in these dose-dependent effects in critically ill patients.[5] In some cases, the variations between individuals can be substantial.[9] Moreover, supposedly predictable dose-dependent dopamine behaviors are only reproducible in patients with normal cardiovascular physiology.[3] Therefore, if you were caring for patients with such physiology, you would not be studying this book.

Why did dopamine fall out of favor?
Once considered first-line vasopressors by the 2008 *Surviving Sepsis Campaign*, dopamine and norepinephrine were evaluated in shock patients in the SOAP II trial.[11] In this randomized controlled trial (RCT), 1679 patients were enrolled, of which 60% were experiencing septic shock. There was no difference in the mortality rate (the primary outcome) after 28 days. The adverse effects were the downfall of dopamine. There was a two-fold increase in cardiac arrhythmias in the dopamine group at 24.1% versus 12.4% ($p < 0.001$). The most common of these arrhythmias was atrial fibrillation, witnessed in one of five patients on dopamine. Another finding was that patients on dopamine had a higher HR for the first 36 hours. However, I wonder whether it meant anything clinically for those patients.

Since then, the *Surviving Sepsis Campaign* has made several strong statements on using dopamine in this patient population. For example, the 2012 Guidelines only recommend dopamine over norepinephrine in patients with relative or absolute bradycardia and those at low risk of tachyarrhythmias.[12] The 2021 update reminds us about the risk of arrhythmia.[13]

What about dopamine in cardiogenic shock?
Dopamine was once the go-to vasopressor for cardiogenic shock patients. Referring again to the SOAP II trial, a subgroup analysis demonstrated that the 280 patients receiving dopamine instead of norepinephrine had a higher mortality rate in patients with cardiogenic shock.[11] Among them, about half were in cardiogenic shock secondary to an acute myocardial infarction (AMI). However, the study did not categorize the outcomes based on the type of cardiogenic shock. Nonetheless, the sample sizes were too small to power and interpret these data appropriately

A 2017 systematic review and meta-analysis of nine studies—including 510 patients with cardiogenic shock—found an association of lower 28-day mortality favoring norepinephrine to dopamine.[14] As anticipated following the SOAP II trial findings, patients receiving dopamine had a higher risk of arrhythmic events. These data included various underlying cardiogenic shock etiologies.

The European Society of Cardiology (ESC) recommends norepinephrine over dopamine in patients with cardiogenic shock requiring vasopressors in their 2016 Guidelines.[15] This recommendation was followed by the American Heart Association (AHA), suggesting that norepinephrine may be the preferred vasopressor in patients with cardiogenic shock within their 2017 Guidelines.[16] Per these data and recommendations, we should not prescribe dopamine for cardiogenic shock patients.

Does dopamine improve renal outcomes?
The short answer is yes if the desired outcome is urine output, as demonstrated in the SOAP II trial.[11] Increased urine output with dopamine has been reported and documented since 1963.[25] However, urine output does not correlate with renal function. Sure, we all cheer when patients hit their hourly urine output goals, but does it change renal outcomes? The urine output increase with dopamine dose was only observed in the first 24 hours. That's it. Subsequently, the playing field became level, with no difference in the fluid balance between the two groups. Most significantly, there was no difference in patients requiring renal support.

A 2000 RCT evaluated 324 patients with early renal dysfunction to receive low-dose dopamine at 2 µg/kg/min or a placebo.[17] There was no difference in any outcomes between both groups. The dopamine did not help. Other reviews suggest that we have zero evidence that renal dose dopamine benefits renal function or patient outcomes with acute kidney injury (AKI).[9,22,23] As a result, data published after those poignant remarks did the "renal dose" dopamine no favors.

A meta-analysis of 24 studies concluded that low-dose dopamine should be eliminated from clinical use to prevent (or treat) renal failure.[26] Furthermore, no kidney-protecting effects were noted in a different systematic review.[27] To put the nail in the coffin, the European Society of Intensive Care Medicine (ESICM) made the highest possible recommendation (Grade 1A) against using low-dose dopamine for protection against AKI.[18]

Can we find an indication of dopamine in the deceased donor population?
While caring for patients diagnosed with death by neurologic criteria, we work closely with organizations assisting in harvesting organs to save other lives. In a specific scenario, the physician working with the organization recommended that I order dopamine for the patient. I was left scratching my head and required some clarification for this idea.

Upon going down the rabbit hole, I found a randomized, open-label trial that provided low-dose dopamine as pretreatment for brain-dead donors, reducing the dialysis requirement after a kidney transplant.[19] Consequently, 4 µg/kg/min of dopamine was provided until the organ cross-clamping. As per the authors, there seemed to be a correlation between the duration of the dopamine infusion and renal outcomes, although the rationale was challenging to narrow down. Overall 264 donors led to 487 kidney transplants. The grafts receiving dopamine had a reduced dialysis need compared to those without getting dopamine at 24.7% versus 35.4%, respectively (p=0.01). These data were preceded by a retrospective database study demonstrating several benefits, including an association with improved long-term graft survival.[28] However, despite these data, there is no formal recommendation to prescribe dopamine in this patient population.[29]

Does dopamine also cause immunosuppression?
Decreased prolactin release and lymphocyte apoptosis have been reported due to dopamine infusions.[20] There are influences on the cytokine network that require clinical studies in patients who are (or are not) critically ill.[21]

Does dopamine blunt the ventilatory drive?
Respiratory responses may be blunted by dopamine.[23,24] Thus, the ventilatory drive response to hypoxemia and hypercapnia can be impaired by depressing the carotid body.

FUN FACTS!
First use of dopamine: The late 1960's.[9]
Onset of action: 5 minutes.[4]
Half-life: 2 minutes.[4]
Duration of action: Less than 10 minutes.[4]
Alternate Name: Intropin

Citations
eddyjoemd.com/dopamine-citations

09: ANGIOTENSIN II

Angiotensin II is the new kid on the block of vasopressors. As with any newcomer, the medical community is still comprehending its role and optimal usage in our armamentarium. While, at the time of this publication, I lack direct experience with angiotensin II, I am optimistic that it can find its niche in our intensive care units. Currently, the landmark trial that forms the cornerstone of our knowledge about angiotensin II is the ATHOS-3 trial.[1] As this medication is relatively new, retrospective observational data is all we have for different subgroups. Hopefully, we will have more soon as most data collected since then is hypothesis-generating. For this chapter, I had the privilege of collaborating with Patrick Wieruszewski, PharmD, an expert in angiotensin II.

What is the mechanism of action of angiotensin II?
Angiotensin II exerts its effects by binding to the angiotensin II type 1 receptor on vascular smooth muscle cells, leading to vasoconstriction.[2] Additionally, it stimulates the release of aldosterone, further influencing blood pressure regulation.

In the MAP = CO x SVR equation, angiotensin II increases the systemic vascular resistance (SVR) to increase the mean arterial pressure (MAP). There is no effect on the cardiac output (CO).

What was the landmark trial for angiotensin II in shock?
The Angiotensin II for the Treatment of High Output Shock (ATHOS-3) trial was the pivotal investigation that led to the FDA approval for angiotensin II's use in septic and other distributive shock states.[1] Conducted by Khanna and colleagues, this randomized controlled trial (RCT) included 344 patients. It was published in the New England Journal of Medicine in 2017. The study contained methodologies aimed at meeting FDA requirements for angiotensin II approval.

Patients requiring greater than 0.2 µg/kg/min of norepinephrine-equivalent dose (NED) vasopressors were randomly assigned to receive angiotensin II or placebo.[1] The primary endpoint was the MAP response at hour 3, requiring the MAP to reach 75 or increase the patient's baseline MAP by at least 10 mmHg. During the trial, 69.9% of patients responded to angiotensin II, achieving the primary endpoint. In contrast, increasing the baseline vasopressor dosage generated a response in only 23.4% of patients. The primary endpoint was met with statistical significance. It is essential to recognize that the ATHOS-3 study employed a MAP goal of 75, higher than the usual 65 aimed for in shock, though this was in line with FDA protocols.

Secondary outcomes in the ATHOS-3 study included cardiovascular and total Sequential Organ Failure Assessment (SOFA) scores, with a statistically significant difference in cardiovascular scores. The use of these scores, in general, has been discussed in published letters amongst colleagues as there are limitations to its interpretation.[3] There was unanimous agreement among experts that the safety profile of angiotensin II requires continued scrutiny. Furthermore, at hour 3, the study demonstrated a statistically significant reduction in the use of other vasopressors when angiotensin II was utilized. No differences were found in all-cause mortality between the groups at day 7 or 28. Several subgroups exhibited potential benefits from angiotensin II, as highlighted in pre-specified and *post hoc* analyses, discussed later in this chapter.

While there was no difference in adverse events, it is noteworthy that using angiotensin II was associated with increased heart rate (HR) during the first six hours after infusion. The package insert also emphasizes an increased risk of thrombosis, a topic we will explore later in this chapter.[2]

Will every patient exhibit a hemodynamic response to angiotensin II?
Not all patients exhibit a reliable hemodynamic response to angiotensin II in refractory shock. For instance, approximately 30.1% of patients did not respond to angiotensin II in the ATHOS-3 trial.[1] Similarly, more recent retrospective studies of 270 and 162 patients demonstrated no-response rates of 33% and 18%, respectively.[4,5] While it may benefit most patients, it is vital to recognize that we should only anticipate a response in some patients when using angiotensin II as a last-ditch effort.

Should we check renin levels to predict who will respond to angiotensin II?
While predicting angiotensin II responders based on renin levels may seem logical, the relationship is more complex. Renin is produced in the kidneys and plays a role in the renin-angiotensin-aldosterone system (RAAS). It cleaves angiotensin I from angiotensinogen, which is then converted into angiotensin II. However, when angiotensin II is abundant, it can inhibit renin release.[6]

A *post hoc* analysis of the ATHOS-3 trial examined renin, angiotensin I, and angiotensin II concentrations in patients and their correlation with outcomes.[7] Patients with renin levels above 173 pg/dL who received angiotensin II exhibited improved outcomes, including decreased 28-day mortality (51% vs. 70%), more frequent liberation from renal replacement therapy by day 7, and more frequent ICU discharge by day 28. Despite the seemingly elevated mortality in these patients, it is essential to note that their median acute physiology and chronic health evaluation (APACHE) II score at baseline indicated a 55% expected mortality.[26] As a reference point, normal plasma renin concentration levels range between 3 and 33 pg/mL.[8]

While checking renin levels may enhance the likelihood of success with such an expensive vasopressor, it is essential to consider the feasibility of such tests in clinical practice. Presently, widespread adoption of renin level assessment is not

76

feasible, although it may hold potential for the future. It is worth noting that plasma renin activity (PRA) is readily available but not interchangeable with direct renin concentration.

What other factors influence angiotensin II responsiveness?
We do not want angiotensin II to work like the cologne *"Sex Panther"* from *Anchorman*. We cannot be spending a significant amount of money on something that, 70% of the time, works all the time (I know the movie says 60%, but Angiotensin II is 70%).

A multi-center retrospective study sought to determine factors contributing to hemodynamic responsiveness to angiotensin II.[4] The study noted that a concomitant vasopressin infusion improved responsiveness to angiotensin II. Patients with lower baseline lactate levels also exhibited a more favorable response. Vasopressin use was associated with a sixfold increase in angiotensin II responsiveness. These findings suggest that central V1 receptor activation may enhance the central pressor effects of angiotensin II.

Could starting angiotensin II earlier in septic shock improve outcomes?
The current practice is to utilize angiotensin II as a salvage therapy in cases of refractory shock due to high costs and lack of familiarity. However, a *post hoc* analysis of the ATHOS-3 trial indicated that earlier initiation of angiotensin II in septic shock patients could lead to improved outcomes.[9] How early? A comparison was conducted of the patients receiving angiotensin II at ≤ 0.25 μg/kg/min or > 0.25 μg/kg/min norepinephrine-equivalent doses (NED) of vasopressors.

Patients receiving angiotensin II at a NED of ≤ 0.25 μg/kg/min exhibited lower mortality compared to the control group, while there was no difference in mortality for patients receiving angiotensin II at NED > 0.25 μg/kg/min. These findings warrant prospective studies to confirm their validity. Similar benefits were reported by Smith *et al.* when angiotensin II was started earlier, with NED < 0.3 μg/kg/min.[5]

Current practice patterns indicate that angiotensin II is typically employed as a fourth-line vasopressor in septic shock.[5] A retrospective observational study found no benefit when angiotensin II was utilized as a third-line vasopressor.[10] Further research on earlier initiation could potentially guide clinical practice, as using angiotensin II as a salvage therapy is not cutting it.

Could angiotensin II help renal outcomes?
Many patients experiencing septic shock also develop renal failure. Unfortunately, evidence supporting vasopressin's role in improving renal outcomes has not been as robust as desired (as observed in VASST and VANISH trials).[11,12] A *post hoc* analysis of 105 patients who developed acute kidney injury (AKI) during the

ATHOS-3 trial aimed to determine whether angiotensin II could contribute to renal function restoration.[13] Among secondary outcomes, there was a statistically significant improvement in the composite of day 7 alive and renal replacement therapy-free at 15% vs. 38% in favor of the angiotensin II group. This scenario raises questions about whether the benefit is associated with specific properties of angiotensin II, reduced catecholamine requirements, or a combination of both. Additional studies are required to provide definitive answers, but given the limited data, it is evident that angiotensin II does not cause harm in this regard.

Can we use angiotensin II in cardiac surgery-related vasoplegia?

Given its ability to improve SVR in distributive shock, angiotensin II could show promise in addressing cardiac surgery-related vasoplegia. A *post hoc* analysis of the ATHOS-3 trial assessed 16 patients who received angiotensin II or a placebo, revealing a much higher response rate in this patient population, with 88.9% of patients (8 of 9) responding positively.[15]

These data, albeit from a small sample, fuel optimism. A double-blind feasibility trial involving sixty patients in this context confirmed the feasibility of conducting a more extensive study. While underpowered to reach definitive conclusions, this study provides hope for angiotensin II's potential in this area.[16] However, a large, randomized, double-blind, placebo-controlled trial would offer the most robust clinical evidence.[17]

Can we use angiotensin II in cardiogenic shock?

Currently, angiotensin II is not recommended for use in cardiogenic shock. Altering afterload (SVR) by administering a vasopressor may adversely affect the struggling heart's ability to maintain adequate CO. The most extensive studies on angiotensin II in cardiogenic shock date back to the early 1960s, involving less than 20 patients compared to norepinephrine.[18,19]

Given the evolving standards of clinical research, it is unfair to scrutinize those studies as we do modern trials, and we should appreciate the pioneering work of their authors. According to Busse et al., one subgroup that might benefit from angiotensin II includes patients on chronic ACE inhibitors in cardiogenic shock.[20] Nevertheless, it is essential to note that the FDA has approved angiotensin II only for septic and other types of distributive shock.[2]

Does angiotensin II affect pulmonary pressures?

Angiotensin receptors have been identified in the pulmonary vascular bed, leading to increased mean pulmonary artery pressure and pulmonary vascular resistance in healthy individuals.[27] However, a retrospective study in patients with mechanical circulatory support demonstrated no increase in mean pulmonary artery pressures.[21] The caveat is that some of these patients were already receiving inotropes and pulmonary vasodilators, potentially mitigating the direct effects of angiotensin II on the pulmonary vascular system.

Vasopressin remains the preferred vasopressor for patients with pulmonary hypertension and right heart failure, as discussed in the *Vasopressin* chapter. Currently, no data supports the use of angiotensin II over vasopressin in patients with pulmonary hypertension, and further investigation is needed to administer angiotensin II in such delicate cases.

Could patients with refractory shock on mechanical circulatory support benefit from angiotensin II?

A retrospective analysis of 14 patients on mechanical circulatory support (MCS) —including VV-ECMO, VA-ECMO, left-ventricular assist device (LVAD), and Impella— who were concurrently receiving vasopressors, revealed that just 36% of patients responded to angiotensin II with an increase in MAP at 3 hours.[22] While it should be recognized as a last-resort measure, angiotensin II may benefit limited patients with MCS. Patients on such support typically have advanced hemodynamic monitoring devices to assist with the careful administration and titration of their vasopressors and inotropes.

What adverse effects should we watch out for?

Patients in the ATHOS-3 trial experienced thromboembolic events at a rate of 12.9%, compared to 5% in the control group.[1] Post-marketing surveillance in Phase IV will aid in determining whether angiotensin II indeed contributes to increased thromboembolic events outside the confines of FDA-defined criteria. In response to this risk, the FDA recommends administering deep vein thrombosis (DVT) prophylaxis.[2,29]

Where are the gaps in our current knowledge of angiotensin II in shock?

As much as we desire more RCTs to determine angiotensin II's place in clinical practice, conducting these trials is more complex. A well-put quote by Paul Young on Twitter/X resonates: *"Before being too critical of any RCT, try doing one. Even simple things are more complicated than they would seem."* Having been a Principal Investigator (PI) for two RCTs, I can attest to the complexity and challenges of conducting clinical trials.

Several gaps remain for future studies to address. These potential research areas include comparing angiotensin II to vasopressin, identifying the optimal timing of its initiation, and formulating guidelines for patient selection in refractory shock.[23] Antonucci *et al.* also highlight the unknowns concerning initiation, potential patient populations who could benefit, the safety profile in patients with myocardial dysfunction, and the peculiar increase in HR observed in patients from the ATHOS-3 trial.[24]

FUN FACTS!
FDA Approval Year: 2017.
Trade Name: *Giapreza*.
Various Names: It is known by several terms, including ANG-2, ANGII, Ang-2, Ang II, angiotonin, and hypertensin.[28]
Half-Life: Angiotensin II has a rapid half-life of less than one minute.[2] This fast elimination rate necessitates careful monitoring by nurses during administration to prevent abrupt hemodynamic changes.
First Literary Mention: Initially named "angiotonin" in 1940, angiotensin II's blood pressure effects were first studied (alongside cocaine) in canine models.[25]
Cost: As of August 31, 2023, per Lexicomp, angiotensin II has a price of $540 for 0.5 mg/mL and $1800 for 2.5 mg/mL

Citations
eddyjoemd.com/angiotensin-2-citations/

80

10: MIDODRINE

Midodrine is a medication we frequently utilize in the ICU setting. It is prescribed to patients who cannot quite get off IV vasopressors for distributive shock and are otherwise doing well. Typically, I initiate a low dose, at 5 mg orally three times a day, and assess the response. From there, I begin titrating up depending on the response. Some playfully call midodrine "*oral phenylephrine*" because they have the exact mechanism of action.

What is the mechanism of action of midodrine?
Midodrine is an orally administered α-1 adrenergic agonist.[1] The α-1 receptors primarily mediate vasoconstriction, and thus, in the context of the MAP = CO x SVR equation, midodrine increases systemic vascular resistance (SVR). There should be no direct effect on cardiac output (CO).

As an inactive prodrug, midodrine is rapidly absorbed in the digestive system with a high bioavailability of 93%.[1] It undergoes enzymatic hydrolysis in the liver to form its active metabolite, desglymidodrine. It is the primary agent that stimulates the α-1 adrenergic receptors, leading to vasoconstriction. Typically, the plasma concentration of desglymidodrine peaks 1-2 hours after ingestion.

Excretion of this active metabolite predominantly occurs through the kidneys, with about 80% being actively secreted.[1] However, in critically ill patients, the pharmacokinetics of midodrine may vary. Factors such as edema of the gastrointestinal tract, which can occur due to excessive volume resuscitation or intestinal vasoconstriction, may alter the absorption and effectiveness of midodrine.

What is the half-life of midodrine?
The half-life of midodrine itself is relatively short, approximately 25 minutes.[1] In contrast, its active metabolite, desglymidodrine, has a longer half-life of about 3-4 hours. This difference in half-life is the basis for the typical dosing regimen of midodrine, which is generally administered three times daily. However, an extended dosing interval of every 6 hours is sometimes also practiced.[2,3]

What could be the benefits of midodrine in the ICU?
Midodrine offers several potential advantages in the ICU setting, primarily stemming from its ability to reduce the use of intravenous (IV) vasopressors:
- **Cost Reduction:** Midodrine can assist in lowering associated costs by reducing reliance on IV vasopressors.
- **Reduced Risk of Infections:** With less requirement for central lines, there is a consequent reduction in the risk of central-line-associated bloodstream infections.

- **Shorter ICU Stays:** As IV vasopressors can be minimized with midodrine, this could lead to shorter lengths of stay in the ICU.

Midodrine Dosing: How Much and How Often?

Initially, when the FDA approved midodrine for treating orthostatic hypotension, the recommended dosage was 10 mg administered three times daily.[1] In clinical trials involving critically ill patients, midodrine has demonstrated efficacy at doses ranging from 5 to 40 mg, taken three times a day.[4]

Various dosing strategies have been recommended in the literature. One common approach is to begin with 20 mg every 8 hours, with the option to incrementally increase the dose by 10 mg daily, up to a maximum of 40 mg every 8 hours.[5] The dose of 40 mg three times a day is the highest dose in a clinical trial.[4]

Other studies have explored more frequent dosage schedules, such as starting with 5 mg every 6 hours, which can be titrated up to 10 mg every 6 hours if needed.[2] This increased dosage frequency of every 6 hours has not raised any significant safety concerns, as indicated by a retrospective trial,[3] and could be an area for further investigation.

What primary side effects should we watch out for in the ICU?

The primary side effect to monitor for in ICU patients receiving midodrine is bradycardia. Numerous studies have discussed its occurrence, with reported incidences varying widely. Some studies indicate a bradycardia incidence of less than 10%,[4,8,10,11,17] while others have found rates as high as 15%.[7,9]

How did midodrine become a staple in our ICUs?

The integration of midodrine into ICU practice began with several observational and retrospective studies. For instance, Levine et al. conducted a prospective observational study in the surgical ICU at Massachusetts General Hospital.[8] They assessed 20 patients on phenylephrine, noting that the average phenylephrine equivalent dose at midodrine initiation was 41.0 ± 33.4 µg/min. Remarkably, 70% of these patients were weaned off vasopressors within the first 24 hours, using a modal dose of 20 mg of midodrine three times daily (p=0.012). Interestingly, the MAP values remained unchanged before and during midodrine administration.

The study by Poveromo et al. expanded the research, evaluating 188 patients receiving vasopressors.[9] The modal dose was 10 mg of midodrine three times daily, but some patients were dosed six times a day. This study highlighted that midodrine could help wean patients off vasopressors in a median of 1.2 days.

Another observational study by Whitson et al. focused on 275 patients, split between those on IV vasopressors alone and those on IV vasopressors plus midodrine.[4] Their results were promising: midodrine plus IV vasopressors shortened the duration of IV vasopressor use (2.9 days vs. 3.8 days, p<0.001), decreased the need for reinstitution of IV vasopressors (5.2% vs. 15%, p=0.007), and resulted in a smaller increase in serum creatinine (0.5 vs. 0.8 mg/dL, p=0.048), as well as a shorter average ICU stay (7.5 days vs. 9.4 days, p=0.017). However, no differences were noted in hospital length of stay or mortality rates. It is also important to note that these patients were already on either stable or decreasing doses of vasopressors.

Another study by Rizvi et al. from the Mayo Clinic, Rochester, retrospectively assessed 1119 patients who were provided with midodrine in the ICU between 2011 and 2016.[7] They found that midodrine use decreased the number of patients on vasopressors after 24 hours (p<0.001) and reduced vasopressor dosages when utilized (p=0.002).

Despite the absence of prospective data, Hammond et al. conducted a systematic review and meta-analysis in 2019 to evaluate midodrine's clinical effects on IV vasopressors in shock patients.[6] Including only three studies, they found no significant decrease in ICU length of stay. The authors suggested that an ideal starting dose might be 20 mg three times a day. In my clinical practice, I often initiate treatment with lower doses.

Observational and retrospective studies are nice, but can we have some RCTs?
The MIDAS and MAVERICK studies stand out as two pivotal randomized controlled trials (RCTs) investigating the use of midodrine in the ICU.[10,11] Let us delve deeper into these studies, particularly the MIDAS trial. This study offered unexpected results that contrasted my positive empirical experiences using midodrine.

MIDAS
The MIDAS trial was a multi-center (USA and Australia) RCT conducted between 2012 and 2019—great job sticking to it by the teams involved.[10] The 132 patients enrolled in this trial were on a single vasopressor for over 24 hours below a specific dose. Patients were randomized in a 1:1 fashion to get either 20 mg of midodrine every 8 hours or a placebo. No titration took place here. In the baseline characteristics of this patient population, only 19.7% of the patients in each group had sepsis. Most of the patients in this study were surgical patients, which differs from how I use it in my practice, which is most commonly in sepsis. The exclusion of patients with renal and liver failure, while understandable from a research perspective, is a point of contention. Previous literature suggests that these patient groups could benefit the most from midodrine.[12-14]

The primary outcome—the median time to discontinuation of IV vasopressors—demonstrated no significant difference between the groups (p=0.62), with 23.5 hours in the midodrine arm and 22.5 hours in the control arm. Additionally, there were no differences in time to discharge readiness from the ICU, median length of stay, hospital length of stay, or ICU readmission rate. Bradycardia was observed in 7.6% of patients in the midodrine group.

The MIDAS trial's results might prompt some to dismiss midodrine as ineffective. The lead author even titled a response in a correspondence series as *"High-dose midodrine is not effective for the treatment of persistent hypotension in the intensive care unit."*[15] However, delving deeper reveals nuances. Santer and Eikermann—in their correspondence—stress that their findings are specific to the surgical ICU setting,[15] suggesting that the results may not be universally applicable to other ICU populations.

Considering the low cost of midodrine compared to ICU care, even a modest benefit could be clinically significant. Medicine, with its inherent uncertainties, often requires individualized approaches. Adjust the dose if midodrine shows no response or adverse effects in a patient. On the other hand, a positive response could warrant the continuation of the treatment. This adaptive approach embodies the art of medicine in balancing empirical evidence with clinical judgment.

MAVERICK
The MAVERICK study—led by Costa-Pinto *et al*. and published in late 2021— explored the use of adjunctive midodrine in patients with vasopressors.[11] The pilot study of 62 patients was cut short due to the emergence of the pandemic, limiting its scope. This open-label trial meant doctors, patients, and staff knew whether midodrine was being administered. A notable aspect of this study was the fixed dosage of midodrine at 10 mg every 8 hours, differing from the variable dosing often utilized in clinical practice.

The outcomes indicated that patients in the midodrine group were weaned off vasopressors slightly faster, though this difference did not reach statistical significance. Similarly, the duration of ICU stays was shorter for the midodrine group, but again, not significantly so. Hospital stay lengths were unaffected by midodrine use. The patient population in this study was diverse, with 40.6% having sepsis and an equal percentage being post-operative patients. Consequently, it becomes complicated to apply these results to specific subgroups.

Given the pilot nature of the study, it is challenging to draw definitive conclusions. Such underpowered studies often provoke debate in the medical community, sometimes leading to premature conclusions about a treatment's effectiveness. The authors acknowledged the risk of a type 2 error due to the small sample size. However, considering the reputation of the study's authors, there is hope that a more comprehensive, non-pilot study from their group will be conducted to evaluate midodrine's efficacy in a broader and more definitive context.

Should we use midodrine after cardiac surgery?

The use of midodrine after cardiac surgery—particularly in patients who have undergone cardiopulmonary bypass (CPB) for valve replacements or grafting—is a topic of ongoing investigation. While the MIDAS trial suggested limited effectiveness of midodrine in post-surgical patients,[10] its role in managing cardiac surgery-related vasoplegia, occurring in 5-25% of CPB patients,[16] warrants further exploration.

A retrospective study at one institution evaluated the practice of using midodrine to treat cardiac surgery-related vasoplegia.[17] In this study of 74 patients on norepinephrine, midodrine was initiated at a median of 27.5 hours post-ICU admission, typically at an initial dose of 10 mg, with rare dose adjustments. Contrary to expectations, the findings could have been more encouraging. Patients receiving midodrine did not exhibit faster weaning from IV vasopressors.

However, more concerning was the observation of higher in-hospital mortality (13.5% vs. 1.4%) and longer ICU stays in the midodrine group. The authors acknowledge significant limitations and potential confounders in their findings, suggesting the need for a prospective RCT to clarify these issues. Currently, no such trials are registered on clinicaltrials.gov, leaving a gap in our understanding of midodrine's efficacy in this specific patient population.

Should we use midodrine in the heart failure population?

The use of midodrine in patients with heart failure presents an intriguing possibility, as demonstrated by a very small study involving chronic systolic heart failure patients.[2] This study included ten patients struggling with medical optimization due to either baseline symptomatic hypotension or symptomatic hypotension induced by their heart failure medications. Intuitively, one might question midodrine use in this context, considering the potential for increased SVR to affect CO in patients with systolic dysfunction adversely.

However, the study's results after six months were surprisingly positive. Patients on midodrine exhibited improvements, allowing for better optimization of medical therapy with ACE inhibitors/ARBs, β-blockers, and aldosterone antagonists like aldactone or eplerenone. Consequently, this led to cardiac remodeling reversal and improved clinical outcomes. Notably, the mean ejection fraction in these patients increased from 24±9.4% to 32.2±9.9% (p<0.001). Additionally, there was a decrease in NYHA class, an improvement in MAP, and a reduction in hospital readmissions. Subsequent research has suggested that α-1 receptor agonists like midodrine may exert adaptive and cardioprotective effects on myocardial tissue.[20,26]

These findings indicate that midodrine could be a valuable adjunct in the management of certain heart failure patients, particularly those who struggle with symptomatic hypotension as a barrier to optimal medical therapy. I would love to see a larger prospective trial that can elaborate on whether this is genuinely beneficial. After all, it would not be a (relatively) expensive trial to conduct. After all, these patients who cannot tolerate their heart failure medications due to hypotension have grim prognoses regardless.

Is midodrine expensive?
Compared to other ICU treatments and resources, midodrine's cost is relatively low. Rizvi et al. reported that the daily cost of midodrine is less than $50.[7] This expenditure is significantly less compared with the daily cost of an ICU bed, which ranges from $3000 to $4000. Given such a disparity in costs, using midodrine, if effective, could lead to considerable savings in healthcare expenditure.

As of July 2023, *UpToDate* provides the following average wholesale prices for midodrine per tablet:
• 2.5 mg: $1.03-1.69
• 5 mg: $1.04-4.49
• 10 mg: $4.84-9.72
Please note that these are not necessarily the prices the hospital or patients pay for the medication.

How long should we wait to observe if midodrine works before quitting?
When considering the effectiveness of midodrine in a patient, expert opinion suggests waiting 24 to 48 hours before determining its efficacy.[19] It is essential to remember that patients may respond differently to various midodrine doses. Like many other medications, midodrine has no universal, one-size-fits-all dosage and response pattern. Therefore, allowing a sufficient period for observation and adjustment of the dosage as needed is crucial in evaluating its impact on each patient.

How should we wean midodrine?
Weaning off midodrine in the ICU and beyond lacks a standardized protocol, yet insights can be gleaned from published experiences and recommendations. One approach—detailed in the correspondence section of CHEST—recommends gradually reducing the midodrine dose by 5 to 10 mg per day until it can be discontinued altogether.[5]

In the context of the MAVERICK trial, a specific weaning protocol was employed. Initially, patients received 10 mg every 8 hours for the first 24 hours following the cessation of IV vasopressors.[11] The dose was then reduced to 7.5 mg every 8 hours for the next 24 hours. Subsequently, the dose was further decreased to 5 mg every 8 hours for another 24 hours. Finally, midodrine was discontinued entirely.

The key point is to remember to discontinue the medication if warranted. As the use of midodrine becomes more prevalent in ICU settings, it is imperative to pay attention to the importance of discontinuing the medication post-discharge. A single-center retrospective study highlighted this oversight, revealing that 67% of patients initiated on midodrine in the ICU were still prescribed it upon discharge.[18] Effective communication is essential to mitigate this issue when transferring a patient from the ICU. In my practice, I either provide a weaning strategy for midodrine to the hospital medicine team or monitor the patient's progress until the medication is safely discontinued.

FUN FACTS!

Discovery of Midodrine: Midodrine (midodrin) was first explored in 1973, with initial experimentation documented in several German publications.[21,22]
FDA Approval: 1996.[23]
FDA-Approved Use: symptomatic orthostatic hypotension.[1]
Off-Label Uses of Midodrine:
• Hepatorenal syndrome.[12]
• Dialysis-induced hypotension.[13]
• Cirrhosis of the liver.[14]
• Post-carotid artery stent placement.[25]
• Advanced heart failure.[2]
• Stunned myocardium.[27]
Brand Name: *Proamatine.*

Citations
eddyjoemd.com/midodrine-citations

11: ISOPROTERENOL

My familiarity with isoproterenol from a practical standpoint was limited at the start of my clinical practice. However, after discovering its role in the ICU, my next logical step was understanding its clinical impact. During this journey, I became aware of its main limitation, which has persisted up to the time of this publication — cost. In my current practice, I only currently utilize isoproterenol to manage symptomatic bradycardia.

What is the mechanism of action of isoproterenol?
Isoproterenol is a potent nonselective β-adrenergic agonist, affecting both β-1 and β-2 receptors. Its effects on these receptors initiate a cascade involving adenylate cyclase. Adenylate cyclase is an enzyme that converts ATP into cAMP, a second messenger that triggers the activation of various proteins. This mechanism ultimately leads to increased heart rate (HR) and contractility. In my practice, I have not utilized isoproterenol for indications associated with contractility.

The β-2 adrenergic receptor activation by isoproterenol in the lungs leads to bronchodilation. Like its impact on heart receptors, β-2 receptors stimulate adenylate cyclase, converting ATP into cAMP and causing bronchodilation. This use was reserved for the operating room in the 1970s.[2] Later, it was also evaluated in the pediatric world for bronchodilation.[3]

β-2 receptors are also found in blood vessels that supply skeletal muscles, uterine tissue, and gastrointestinal smooth muscle. While isoproterenol's vasodilatory effect is observed in coronary and cutaneous vessels, it is more pronounced in muscular vessels.[4] However, this scenario cannot discount its influence on coronary vessels, where it triggers a coronary vasodilator response by stimulating both vascular and myocardial β receptors. In the literature, the direct vascular effect predominates.[5]

In the MAP = CO x SVR equation, isoproterenol enhances cardiac output (CO) by increasing the HR and stroke volume (SV). A quick reminder that CO = HR x SV and that SV has three components: preload, afterload, and contractility.

Where is isoproterenol utilized in the clinical setting?
Despite its strong inotropic and systemic vasodilatory impact, isoproterenol's utility in clinical practice is constrained due to its chronotropic effects.[7] Consequently, its primary indication is treating bradycardia. Moreover, it is listed alongside other therapies in the American Heart Association (AHA) recommendations for bradycardia, including atropine, dopamine, dobutamine, and epinephrine.[8] Other indications include complete heart block,[9] premature

labor,[10] and anesthesia-related bronchospasm.[2] It is also utilized in certain cardiac electrophysiology studies.

Why isn't isoproterenol the first line for symptomatic bradycardia?

Isoproterenol is often utilized in the Cardiac ICU due to its chronotropic effect, meaning its ability to increase HR. A clinical example can be a patient presenting with certain symptomatic bradycardia. In these cases, initial treatments include dopamine or epinephrine, as the ACLS guidelines recommend.[1] If these treatments are ineffective, and we cannot place a transvenous pacemaker, we may initiate isoproterenol. However, due to its high cost at the time of this publication, we usually do not utilize isoproterenol as the first-line chronotropic agent.

When was isoproterenol first utilized in human clinical trials?

A thorough exploration of *PubMed* reveals several relevant studies published as early as 1947.[11] Both bench and animal-based research studies have examined isoproterenol's impact on the lungs, heart, kidneys, adrenal glands, aorta, and uterus. A remarkable historical event is the earliest known usage of an artificial pacemaker in a patient who suffered from severe *Adams-Stokes* syndrome and complete heart block. Isoproterenol was prescribed to support this patient, although the outcome was unfortunately fatal due to left heart failure.[12] Even after a decade since the first publications on isoproterenol, this medication's exact mechanism of action and impacts were still being figured out in 1959.[13]

Why is isoproterenol so expensive?

Isoproterenol prices dramatically increased 70-fold from 2012 to 2015.[14] This period aligns with my residency and commencement of fellowship, which is likely why I had limited training on isoproterenol. This massive cost surge resulted in a reduction in its utilization as an alternative option. Hopefully, these pricing issues will be resolved soon.

What are the contraindications of isoproterenol?

While some contraindications may seem self-evident, it is imperative to stress that isoproterenol should not be administered to patients with tachyarrhythmias, tachycardia, or angina. The rationale behind these contraindications include isoproterenol elevating myocardial oxygen consumption while reducing coronary perfusion, thus posing a risk of inducing an acute myocardial infarction (AMI).[15] An animal study demonstrated increased myocardial infarct size when providing isoproterenol. Additionally, the package insert advises against prescribing isoproterenol to patients with digitalis intoxication due to documented instances of precipitated ectopic rhythms and electrocardiographic deterioration in 1962.[16,20]

Can we use isoproterenol for sepsis?

No, we should not use isoproterenol for sepsis. The *Surviving Sepsis Campaign* does not list it as an option.[17] Despite its limited application, isoproterenol was once regarded as an alternative to dobutamine in specific scenarios. It was introduced alongside norepinephrine in 14 septic shock patients with SvO2 levels below 70%, leading to an improvement in key parameters, including cardiac index, stroke index, and SvO2.[18] However, no ongoing studies have been conducted to compare isoproterenol to dobutamine directly.

How should we dose isoproterenol?

For those considering isoproterenol for shock, the package insert recommends an infusion rate of 0.5 to 5 µg/min.[20] For heart block, a bolus and subsequent infusion are recommended, however, I have not needed to provide a bolus. The initial bolus is listed as 0.02 - 0.06 mg. This is followed by an infusion at 5 µg/min. I have noted institutions started at 2 µg/min instead. This therapy acts immediately and offers alternative routes of administration, including intramuscular, subcutaneous, and intracardiac dosing, although my personal experience is limited in this regard.

FUN FACTS!

Brand Name: *Isuprel*. This name has historical significance, as earlier publications from the 1940s and 1950s often referred to the drug by its brand name rather than its generic name in their titles.[11,12,19]

Alternate Name: Isoprenaline.

Historical Uses: I was unaware of an intriguing indication until I conducted in-depth research while writing this book—*i.e.,* using isoproterenol for pulmonary hypertension.[6] Although my conversations with my pulmonologist colleagues did not reveal this as a currently employed therapy, it is an interesting aspect of isoproterenol's clinical history.

Citations

eddyjoemd.com/isoproterenol-citations

12: DOBUTAMINE

According to a European Society of Intensive Care Medicine survey, dobutamine is the first-line inotrope for enhancing cardiac pump function for 82% of its members.[1] This consensus has led to a strong recommendation for its use as the first-line inotrope. The preference for dobutamine is partly due to its short half-life of less than two minutes, allowing for rapid action and easier titration by nursing staff.[2] In clinical practice, the choice of inotrope often reflects personal experience. However, I advocate for a patient-centric approach, selecting the inotrope based on individual patient needs.

What is the mechanism of action of dobutamine?
Dobutamine primarily stimulates β-1-adrenergic receptors, enhancing myocardial contractility, and to a lesser extent, α-1-adrenergic receptors, which can influence vascular tone.[3,4] Its affinity for β-2-adrenergic receptors is weaker, described as 10-fold less than for β-1.[5]

In the context of the MAP = CO x SVR equation, dobutamine increases cardiac output (CO) by augmenting stroke volume (SV) and, to a lesser extent, heart rate, both consequences of β-1 receptor stimulation. Although α-1 receptor stimulation typically leads to vasoconstriction, dobutamine can paradoxically cause vasodilation, possibly due to β-2 receptor effects, thus decreasing systemic vascular resistance (SVR).[2,6,7]

The dose-dependent effects on α-1 receptors will be discussed shortly, underscoring the variability of dobutamine's impact on mean arterial pressure (MAP). The net effect on MAP could be variable using dobutamine as the CO and SVR effects could balance themselves out.[3,6] In my practice, these patients undergo hemodynamic monitoring to assess the CO and SVR. Clinicians may need to add norepinephrine due to the unpredictability of the SVR.[2]

Are dobutamine's effects dose-dependent?
Dobutamine's influence on SVR and heart rate (HR) is indeed dose-dependent.[8] Beginning with its variable effects on SVR, at lower doses (less than 5 μg/kg/min), a decrease in SVR is typically observed.[4] In the mid-range, up to 15 μg/kg/min, dobutamine does not significantly impact SVR. However, at higher doses (greater than 15 μg/kg/min), vasoconstriction becomes the predominant effect.

Regarding the HR, dobutamine's effect also varies with dosage.[9] Doses up to 5 μg/kg/min generally do not alter the heart rate. A notable increase in heart rate begins at doses around 7.5 μg/kg/min,[20] and at doses higher than 10 μg/kg/min, there is a risk of inducing tachycardia.[9]

Is dobutamine effective in optimizing patients with severe decompensated heart failure?

In the management of severe decompensated heart failure, where patients are not in cardiogenic shock, inotropes like dobutamine are often utilized to improve cardiac function and return their physiology back onto the Frank-Starling curve. However, what does the evidence say about this practice commonly occurring today? A 2012 systematic review and meta-analysis, which included 14 studies and 672 patients, found no significant mortality benefit when dobutamine was utilized compared to a placebo.[12]

Other outcomes, such as hospital length of stay, incidence of renal failure, or symptom relief, might offer more insight into dobutamine's effectiveness. However, these were not evaluated in this paper. Demonstrating a mortality benefit in hemodynamically stable heart failure patients can be particularly challenging. In my opinion, these data should not influence our management.

Are dobutamine and β-blockers compatible in managing decompensated heart failure?

Managing decompensated heart failure in patients already on β-blockers presents a clinical challenge. While β-blockers are known to reduce mortality in such patients, as evidenced by a retrospective study of 3817 patients, they also pose the risk of further lowering their marginal MAP.[10] Note that these patients were not in cardiogenic shock.

The choice of inotrope in these patients can be influenced by the specific β-blocker they are on. For instance, Metra *et al.* found that carvedilol, a non-selective β-blocker, significantly attenuated the effects of dobutamine on CO, HR, and SV.[13] In contrast, metoprolol, a selective β-blocker, had a minor impact on dobutamine's hemodynamic responses.

To overcome the dampening effects of non-selective β-blockers like carvedilol, higher dobutamine doses (15-20 μg/kg/min) may be required, as highlighted by Lowes *et al.*[14] However, this comes with the risk of hypertension.[15] In cases where a patient is chronically on a non-selective β-blocker, milrinone might be a preferable inotropic choice.

How do dobutamine and levosimendan compare in the treatment of cardiogenic shock or low cardiac output syndrome?

According to a 2020 Cochrane Systematic Review, when treating cardiogenic shock or low cardiac output syndrome, there appears to be no significant difference between dobutamine and levosimendan regarding all-cause short-term mortality, all-cause long-term mortality, and MAP.[16] However, the review did highlight certain advantages of levosimendan over dobutamine. These include improvements in cardiac index and a reduction in pulmonary capillary wedge pressure.

How does dobutamine differ from isoproterenol in its cardiac effects?

Dobutamine and isoproterenol, while both being inotropes, exhibit distinct effects on HR and peripheral vascular resistance. Dobutamine, known for its potent inotropic action, causes a lesser increase in HR (chronotropy) and a smaller reduction in peripheral vascular resistance than isoproterenol. Importantly, dobutamine primarily boosts CO by increasing SV. In contrast, isoproterenol raises CO chiefly by elevating HR and inducing a more pronounced decrease in SVR.

How does dobutamine affect pulmonary artery pressures?

The response of pulmonary artery pressures to dobutamine is a prime example of the intricacies involved in the advanced hemodynamic management of critically ill patients. The effect of dobutamine on these pressures is only partially predictable and remains a subject of ongoing debate. Research from as far back as the 1970s has produced mixed results.[3,17]

Some studies indicate a decrease in pulmonary artery pressure following dobutamine administration, while others report no significant change or increase.[3,17] This inconsistency in data results in a certain level of uncertainty regarding dobutamine's impact on pulmonary artery pressures. On a more definitive note, milrinone has been recognized for its more reliable effects in reducing pulmonary artery pressures.[18,19]

Does the combination of epinephrine and dobutamine result in a synergistic effect?

It might be assumed that combining epinephrine with dobutamine would synergistically boost CO. However, this expectation does not align with reality, as evidenced by a 1998 study.[20] Contrary to the anticipated additive effect of these drugs on CO, the study observed what was termed 'pseudoantagonism' in a cardiac surgery cohort.

This surprising outcome implies that the combined use of epinephrine and dobutamine might not necessarily lead to improved therapeutic effects and warrants careful observation for hemodynamic and cardiovascular impacts. While this finding relates explicitly to cardiac surgery patients, it raises pertinent questions about the effectiveness of this drug combination in other types of cardiogenic shock. More comprehensive research in these areas is, however, still needed.

Does dobutamine become less effective over time?

Contrary to a common pharmacological belief that continuous receptor activation ensures sustained drug efficacy, dobutamine presents a notable exception. Prolonged usage of dobutamine can lead to tachyphylaxis, a phenomenon where the drug's effectiveness diminishes over time.[6] This reduction in efficacy has been observed in studies where patients demonstrated a decline in the initially improved hemodynamics.[20] Notably, a 1980 study involving 20 patients documented hemodynamic tolerance emerging after 72 hours of dobutamine use.[22] In instances of such tolerance, increasing the dose to achieve the desired effect is often recommended.[20] However, to reduce the risk of tachyphylaxis, it is advised to keep the dobutamine dosage at or below 5 µg/kg/min.[25]

Is dobutamine an acceptable choice for patients with septic shock?
According to the *Surviving Sepsis Campaign*, dobutamine, along with epinephrine, is frequently employed in treating septic shock.[23] Notably, up to 20% of patients with septic shock develop sepsis-induced cardiomyopathy (SIC).[24] It is essential to consider the hemodynamic response variability of the SVR discussed earlier, as dobutamine can cause vasodilation, potentially exacerbating the distributive shock in these patients. While there is a lack of studies focusing solely on dobutamine use in septic shock, subsequent sections will explore its combined use with norepinephrine.

In cases of septic shock with low cardiac output, should we use dobutamine with norepinephrine or epinephrine alone?
It is worth mentioning again that approximately 20% of patients with septic shock also develop SIC.[24] Our typical approach involves initiating norepinephrine and adding vasopressin as the second-line agent in septic shock. However, this scenario can lead to suboptimal treatment in one in five patients if SIC is not identified and addressed suitably. It is vital to implement mechanisms for identifying SIC to customize treatment accordingly. Therefore, a pivotal question is whether to add dobutamine to norepinephrine or to switch to epinephrine in such scenarios.

The 2007 CATS trial offers some insights into this dilemma. It illustrated no significant difference in various outcomes between patients treated with either epinephrine (alone or combined with dobutamine) and norepinephrine for septic shock patients with low cardiac index.[26] However, the study observed more frequent transient elevations in lactate levels in the epinephrine group, with no notable differences in the rate of serious adverse effects.

Given that norepinephrine is the recommended first-line vasopressor in septic shock patients, according to the SSC, adding dobutamine to an already-running norepinephrine infusion has a practical advantage. This approach could minimize waste and simplify management. However, the potential drawback could be limited IV access or pump availability for managing two distinct infusions. Thus, the choice between adding dobutamine or switching to epinephrine should be based on clinical efficacy and practical logistics in each patient's unique situation.

Why should we exercise caution in administering dobutamine to patients with atrial fibrillation?
Administering dobutamine to patients who have atrial fibrillation can be risky as it may escalate to atrial fibrillation with rapid ventricular rate (RVR).[11,15] This heightened risk is attributed to dobutamine's propensity to increase the velocity of conduction through the atrioventricular node. Therefore, in cases where a patient already presents with atrial fibrillation with RVR, initiating treatment with digoxin prior to dobutamine is advisable to mitigate these risks.[1]

FUN FACTS!
Alternative Names: *Dobutrex*
Origin Story: dobutamine is derived from isoproterenol.[5]
Half-life and Onset: Half-life is 2 minutes.[11] The onset of action is 1-2 minutes, but it could take 10 minutes to observe the peak effect.[11]
Contraindications: patients with Hypertrophic Obstructive Cardiomyopathy.[11]
Dosing Range: 2-20 µg/kg/min.[2,27,28,29]
Maximum Dose in the Literature: 40 µg/kg/min[8] or 50 µg/kg/min.[15]

Citations
eddyjoemd.com/dobutamine-citations

13: MILRINONE

Milrinone, commonly utilized in Cardiac and Cardiothoracic ICUs, is an inodilator — a term blending 'inotrope' and 'vasodilator.' This means milrinone increases cardiac output (CO) through inotropic effects and decreases systemic vascular resistance (SVR) through its dilator properties, impacting the mean arterial pressure (MAP) equation: MAP = CO x SVR.

It is crucial to use milrinone cautiously in patients with distributive shock, where SVR is already low. Further reducing SVR in these cases can be detrimental. In clinical practice, milrinone often necessitates concurrent use of norepinephrine. I call these two 'best friends'. This observation is not unique to my experience, as others have noted similar findings.[1]

In this chapter and the next, we will also encounter enoximone, another phosphodiesterase 3 inhibitor. The medical literature often regards enoximone as functionally similar to milrinone from a mechanistic perspective.[2]

What is the mechanism of action of milrinone?
Milrinone operates differently compared to catecholamine-based inotropes like dobutamine. While dobutamine activates β-receptors, increasing cyclic adenosine monophosphate (cAMP), milrinone elevates cAMP by inhibiting phosphodiesterase 3 (PDE3). This action effectively mimics β-1 and β-2 receptor activation without directly stimulating these receptors.[3]

This rise in cAMP yields multiple cardiac effects: enhanced contractility (positive inotropy), improved diastolic myocardial relaxation (lusitropy), and better atrioventricular conduction (dromotropy).[1] These effects stem from increased intracellular calcium concentration, which bolsters contractility and hastens myocardial relaxation.[4]

Conversely, milrinone's impact extends to vascular smooth muscles. Here, the elevated cAMP levels induce vasodilation in arterial and venous circulation, contrasting with its effects on cardiac tissue. This vasodilation results in a decrease in SVR.[1,4]

What are some advantages of milrinone over other inotropes?
Milrinone offers several advantages over other inotropes, particularly in the context of cardiogenic shock and post-cardiac surgery scenarios. One key benefit is its dual action: increasing CO and decreasing SVR. This vasodilation, rather than being a mere side effect, is a valuable feature, especially for patients in the early stages of cardiogenic shock who often exhibit elevated SVR as a compensatory response to decreased CO. Milrinone effectively addresses both issues, improving hemodynamic parameters as evidenced by improved readings

on hemodynamic monitoring devices. Its ability to reduce pulmonary vascular resistance (PVR) also contributes to its recognition as a highly useful inotrope for managing low output syndrome after cardiac surgery.[5]

Another significant advantage of milrinone is its lack of effect on heart rate (HR). Unlike other inotropes, milrinone does not increase myocardial oxygen consumption, an essential consideration in managing patients with limited cardiac reserve. This was highlighted in a 1986 study that compared milrinone and dobutamine, demonstrating similar improvements in cardiac index between the two drugs but without increased myocardial oxygen consumption often associated with dobutamine.[6] This characteristic of milrinone makes it particularly beneficial for patients where increasing HR and myocardial oxygen demand would be detrimental.

Why are milrinone and right heart failure friends?
Milrinone establishes itself as a particularly effective option in managing right heart failure. Its advantages in right heart failure are highlighted through various studies:

- A 1986 study demonstrated milrinone's ability to significantly reduce right atrial pressures in patients with severe congestive heart failure, an advantage not as pronounced with dobutamine.[6]
- In 1996, research demonstrated that milrinone significantly improved pulmonary artery systolic and diastolic pressures. While improvements in PVR and mean pulmonary artery pressures were also observed with milrinone, these were not statistically significant in this study.[7]
- A 1997 study focused on patients with pulmonary hypertension secondary to severe heart failure. It found that boluses of milrinone consistently decreased PVR, a crucial factor in managing right heart failure.[8]
- In 2009, milrinone was compared with sildenafil in patients awaiting heart transplants. Both drugs similarly affected PVR, but milrinone also decreased pulmonary capillary wedge pressure due to its inotropic effect.[9]

These studies underscore milrinone's superiority in managing patients with right ventricular dysfunction over dobutamine. There are additional studies, but I would rather not bore you further. Its specific action on reducing PVR and other related pressures makes it a valuable tool in treating right heart failure.

How should milrinone be administered?
Administering a bolus dose of milrinone requires careful consideration. The recommended dosage is 50 µg/kg over 10 minutes,[14] but it is crucial to proceed cautiously. While some studies indicate that such a bolus dose does not significantly impact systemic arterial pressure,[8] it is wise to be prepared for potential hypotension. Seneca aptly said, *"Luck is what happens when*

preparation meets opportunity." Therefore, having norepinephrine, milrinone's *'best friend,'* nearby is prudent in case of a sudden drop in blood pressure.

The hemodynamic effects of a milrinone bolus are described as reaching their peak 5 to 10 minutes post-infusion, emphasizing that immediate effects should not be expected.[8,22] It is important to monitor the patient and adjust treatment based on their response after this period.

Regarding continuous infusions, starting doses of 0.5 µg/kg/hr have been observed in various clinical trials.[10,11] The DOREMI trial, a recent randomized controlled trial (RCT) of dobutamine versus milrinone, employed initial dose ranges of 0.125, 0.25, 0.375, 0.5, and greater than 0.5 µg/kg/min. Some sources suggest that the dose can be increased to 1.0 µg/kg/min, depending on the patient's response and tolerance.[4] As with any drug, individual patient factors and clinical judgment are critical in determining the optimal dosing strategy.

Do we need to provide a loading dose of milrinone?
The administration of a 50 µg/kg over 10 minutes loading dose of milrinone is not a necessity. While it is common to anticipate a delay before observing significant hemodynamic effects from milrinone, typically around 30 minutes, the need for a loading dose is not universally required. This approach is supported by a small trial which revealed that patients who started on an infusion without a loading dose experienced similar outcomes to those who received a bolus.[12] This finding suggests that the infusion alone can effectively achieve the desired hemodynamic impact, allowing for a more gradual onset of action and potentially reducing the risk of sudden hemodynamic changes.

Why is knowing the half-life of milrinone necessary?
Milrinone, distinct in its pharmacologic profile, boasts a longer half-life than many of its inotropic counterparts. This extended duration of action, averaging between 2 to 3 hours,[13,14] makes it suitable for patients with adrenergic receptor desensitization or those accustomed to prolonged β-agonist therapy.

The importance of milrinone's half-life bears direct implications for patient care. Clinicians and nurses, often more familiar with inotropes of shorter half-lives, must tread carefully with milrinone's titration. Rapid weaning risks a sudden withdrawal of hemodynamic support — akin to pulling the rug from under the patients' feet — potentially destabilizing them.

Should we be cautious about milrinone in renal failure?
Milrinone is predominantly excreted via the urine, and in the context of renal impairment, this could lead to prolonged drug action. Adjusting the maintenance dose is warranted in such cases.[5] Patients with renal failure may experience an extended half-life of milrinone, potentially increasing from the usual 2 to 3 hours to about 4 to 6 hours. This prolongation raises concerns about drug accumulation

and the risk of prolonged adverse effects, such as arrhythmias.[13] The package insert advises dose modification in patients with renal impairment.[14]

However, a retrospective cohort study published in March 2023 presents a nuanced perspective.[15] This study, focusing on patients who underwent cardiac surgery and had renal dysfunction, did not alter milrinone dosing based on creatinine clearance despite the patients receiving weight-based dosing. Intriguingly, among the 197 patients included, there was no observed increase in arrhythmias. While these findings are retrospective and thus warrant cautious interpretation, they suggest that milrinone may not necessarily need to be avoided in patients with renal dysfunction.

Does the Use of β-Blockers Influence the Efficacy of Milrinone?
In the *Dobutamine* chapter, we delved into how non-selective β-blockers like carvedilol modify the effects of inotropes.[16] Extending those discussions, it is noteworthy that the advantages of phosphodiesterase (PDE) inhibitors, such as milrinone, are not diminished when utilized alongside β-blockers. For instance, combining enoximone (another PDE inhibitor) with carvedilol increased stroke volumes and higher cardiac indices, illustrating a synergistic effect. However, caution is warranted. This combination also intensified the reduction in MAP and SVR in some patients, indicating potential risks. Administering milrinone with β-blockers may offer a therapeutic advantage by mitigating the pro-arrhythmic effects of milrinone, a notable concern with inodilators.[4]

Can we combine milrinone with β-agonists?
In certain challenging clinical scenarios, patients may require additional inotropic support beyond what β-agonists like dobutamine can offer. The unique mechanism of milrinone, which does not directly interact with β-adrenergic receptors, becomes particularly relevant here. This distinction is crucial when considering adding catecholamine inopressors such as norepinephrine or epinephrine to a patient already receiving dobutamine. These combinations may not provide the desired therapeutic effect due to overlapping β-adrenergic activity.

Research, especially in cardiac surgery patients, has shed light on this. Studies examining the synergistic effects of milrinone (with its analogs like enoximone and amrinone) and dobutamine suggest benefits in specific contexts.[17,18] However, it is essential to approach this combination cautiously. Evidence from an observational trial indicated that patients requiring two inotropes, such as a β-agonist and milrinone, might experience worse outcomes.[19] This finding highlights the complexity and risk associated with polypharmacy in cardiac care.

Does milrinone improve outcomes in decompensated heart failure?
This question was central to two pivotal studies: the Prospective Randomised Milrinone Survival Evaluation (PROMISE) trial and the Outcomes of Prospective

Trial of Intravenous Milrinone for Exacerbations of Chronic Heart Failure (OPTIME-CHF).

The PROMISE trial aimed to determine the long-term impact of milrinone on survival in chronic heart failure patients.[20] In this 1991 study, 1088 patients were randomized to receive either oral milrinone or a placebo and followed for six months. The outcomes were disheartening; those on milrinone demonstrated a 28% increase in all-cause mortality and a 38% increase in cardiovascular mortality. The mortality rate was even higher (53%) in patients with Class IV heart failure. Additionally, there were more hospitalizations and increased instances of hypotension and syncope. These results may explain why many of us are unfamiliar with oral milrinone.

In the OPTIME-CHF trial, 951 patients with systolic heart failure exacerbations who were not in cardiogenic shock were assigned either milrinone or placebo.[10] Milrinone was infused for 48 hours. This trial also yielded unfavorable results, showing more sustained hypotension (10.7% vs. 3.2%, NNT=13.3) and arrhythmias (8.5% vs. 1.5%, NNT=14.3) in the milrinone group, including atrial fibrillation, atrial flutter, ventricular tachycardia, and ventricular fibrillation. The groups had no significant differences in length of stay, inpatient mortality, 60-day mortality, or readmission rates. Consequently, the routine use of milrinone in chronic heart failure exacerbations is not recommended.

Furthermore, a *post hoc* analysis of the OPTIME-CHF data revealed that patients with ischemic heart failure etiology fared worse on milrinone, with higher rates of death or rehospitalization at 60 days compared to their non-ischemic counterparts (38.7% vs. 31.5%, p=0.02). This suggests an increased risk associated with milrinone in certain patient subsets.

What key adverse effects should we watch for?
Certain adverse effects of administering milrinone merit close monitoring. Hypotension is a notable concern, particularly in patients who already present with low systemic vascular resistance (SVR) or hypovolemia. Additionally, arrhythmias are another significant adverse effect associated with milrinone, as is common with most inotropes.

FUN FACTS!
FDA-Approval: 1987.[14]
Alternate names and related drugs: *Primacor* (trade name).[14] Enoximone is also a PDEi unavailable in the US. *Amrinone* (the parent drug) has a 10% rate of thrombocytopenia caused by reversible bone marrow suppression.[4] Milrinone was synthesized after a modification to this drug.

Citations
eddyjoemd.com/milrinone-citations

14: MILRINONE VS. DOBUTAMINE

The debate over the superiority of milrinone versus dobutamine continues to be a significant issue in both clinical practice and medical literature. In this chapter, we delve into the (limited) data contributing to this debate, highlighting the importance of individual patient characteristics and tolerance for adverse effects in choosing the appropriate treatment for decompensated heart failure, cardiogenic shock, or low cardiac output syndrome (LCOS) post-cardiac surgery.

Cardiogenic Shock: Is There a Clear Winner?
While the landmark trial comparing milrinone and dobutamine demands attention, it is crucial to acknowledge the plethora of preceding trials that have shaped current practices. A 2019 systematic review and meta-analysis comparing milrinone and dobutamine in LCOS and/or cardiogenic shock was limited by the presence of only one randomized controlled trial (RCT), including just 36 patients.[15]

The DOREMI trial, published in the New England Journal of Medicine in 2021, randomized 192 patients in cardiogenic shock to receive either dobutamine or milrinone.[1] This trial is particularly intriguing due to clinicians and institutions' apparent bias towards one inotrope over another.

These patients were notably sick, with over 80% in SCAI shock stage C and a median ejection fraction of 25%. Interestingly, only 23 of the 192 patients had a pulmonary artery catheter (PAC) at enrollment, contrasting the heavy reliance on PAC in my practice for managing cardiogenic shock.

The trial reported no significant differences in a comprehensive primary and secondary outcomes list. This includes detailed subgroup analyses and arrhythmia occurrence, noted in about 50% of patients in both groups.[2] Despite the faster metabolism of dobutamine (half-life of 2 minutes) compared to milrinone (> 2 hours), there was no significant difference in length of hospital stay or total time receiving inotropes. This highlights the necessity of personalized management in selecting the optimal inotrope.

For those seeking further insights, the DOREMI-2 trial is currently underway, aiming to enroll 346 patients for a more robust comparison (NCT05267886).

Cardiogenic Shock Patients on Carvedilol: Is There a Clear Winner?
As discussed in previous chapters on *Dobutamine* and *Milrinone*, it is advisable to administer milrinone to patients on non-selective β-blockers like carvedilol based on studies referenced in the respective chapters.[3,4]

Cardiac Surgery Patients: Is There a Clear Winner?
Patients emerging from cardiac surgery with low cardiac output syndrome (LCOS) present a critical decision point for inotrope selection.[5] Here's a snapshot of what various studies have revealed:
• 1990: Same clinical effect and no significant difference in all-cause short-term mortality between dobutamine and enoximone groups, with the dobutamine group experiencing longer ICU stays.[6] Note: This study, published only in French, provided limited data from the abstract. I cannot read in that language.
• 1990: No significant difference between dobutamine and enoximone regarding cardiac index and pulmonary capillary wedge pressure was demonstrated.[7] Patients receiving enoximone were observed to have less myocardial oxygen consumption and lower blood pressure.
• 2001: Comparing dobutamine and milrinone demonstrated similar effects on the cardiac index, pulmonary capillary wedge pressure, and MAP.[8] However, dobutamine was associated with more hypertension and atrial fibrillation, while milrinone had more incidences of bradycardia. This study on inotropes for cardiogenic shock is highlighted in the Cochrane Review.[9]
• 2018: An RCT including patients with mitral stenosis and pulmonary hypertension undergoing mitral valve replacement compared milrinone with a combination of dobutamine and nitroglycerin.[10] Milrinone demonstrated superior efficacy in reducing mean pulmonary artery pressure and pulmonary capillary wedge pressure.
• 2019: This study, predominantly involving cardiac surgery patients, noted more arrhythmias with dobutamine and more hypotension with milrinone, although their overall effects were similar.[11]
• 2023: A systematic review and meta-analysis attempted to consolidate these and other data but found most fell into the 'high risk of bias' category, underscoring the need for personalized management.[12]

These studies, with their small patient numbers and varying surgical procedures, reinforce the importance of a tailored approach in the ICU.

Patients Awaiting a Heart Transplant: Is There a Clear Winner?
Determining the superior agent is crucial for hospitalized patients awaiting a heart transplant. A 2003 study revealed no difference in outcomes between milrinone and dobutamine, except for cost, with milrinone being more expensive.[13] However, current pricing information is beyond the scope of this book.

Patients on Palliative Inotropes: Is there a clear winner?
The choice of inotrope becomes crucial in palliative care, specifically for patients unsuitable for heart transplants or left ventricular assist devices (LVADs). Often managed at home, these patients may require a peripherally inserted central catheter (PICC) line for continuous infusion of either milrinone or dobutamine. It provides us something to offer these patients who are otherwise terminal.

A 2022 study investigated this scenario in a cohort of 248 patients.[14] Despite the high mortality rates inherent to this patient group, the study revealed a significant difference in survival outcomes between the two medications. Patients on milrinone demonstrated a notably lower mortality rate (58%) than those on dobutamine (84%). This difference was statistically significant (p<0.001), with a number needed to treat (NNT) of 3.8, indicating that for every 3.8 patients treated with milrinone instead of dobutamine, one additional life could be saved.

Do we have a winner?
This chapter's journey through various clinical scenarios and study findings reiterates the importance of considering individual patient characteristics, underlying conditions, hemodynamic data, and the specific clinical context when deciding between milrinone and dobutamine. The high variability in patient responses and the absence of a one-size-fits-all solution highlight our need to stay informed, flexible, and patient-centric in our approach.

Citations
eddyjoemd.com/milrinone-vs-dobutamine

15: LEVOSIMENDAN

Levosimendan remains outside the realm of my clinical experience. Currently, it is not FDA-approved and unavailable in the United States. However, given the evolving nature of pharmacotherapy and drug approvals, there is potential for its introduction into the U.S. healthcare system in the future. This section provides an overview of levosimendan, preparing US clinicians for its possible emergence in clinical practice. As per PubMed, the academic interest in levosimendan is evident, with over 80 publications annually since 2006, underscoring its importance in the medical field.

What is the mechanism of action of levosimendan?

Levosimendan, recognized for its inotropic and vasodilatory properties, functions as a myofilament calcium-sensitizing drug. It enhances cardiac output (CO) by sensitizing the myocardium to calcium through binding to cardiac troponin.[1,2] Additionally, its vasodilatory effects are facilitated by opening ATP-sensitive potassium channels in vascular smooth muscle, leading to smooth muscle relaxation.[3]

Notably, levosimendan presents an advantage over catecholamines. It can increase contractility without a corresponding increase in myocardial oxygen demand, a feature that has led to its classification as 'cardioprotective' in the medical literature.[3,4] Furthermore, it does not impair diastolic relaxation, an essential aspect of heart function.[5]

Regarding hemodynamics, levosimendan impacts the equation MAP = CO x SVR by increasing CO through augmented stroke volume (SV) while decreasing systemic vascular resistance (SVR).

Has levosimendan been studied in cardiac surgery patients?

Patients undergoing cardiac surgery may experience low-cardiac-output syndrome (LCOS), necessitating inotropes or mechanical circulatory support to manage reduced cardiac output.[2]

In recent years, levosimendan has been explored as a prophylactic treatment for those at risk of LCOS. Three randomized controlled trials (RCTs) in 2017 —LEVO-CTS, LICORN, and CHEETAH—investigated its efficacy.[6,7,8] However, the results of these studies, as analyzed by Welker et al., have not been conclusively favorable.[2] For instance, the CHEETAH trial was prematurely halted due to futility. Such outcomes highlight the importance of nuanced interpretation in clinical studies, especially considering variables like the median preoperative ejection fraction (EF), which was 50% in the CHEETAH trial.

Despite no observed difference in mortality and several other outcomes with levosimendan use, Welker *et al.* suggest that specific patient demographics — namely, those with an EF ≤ 25%, advanced age over 65, and female sex — might still benefit from its prophylactic use to prevent LCOS.[2]

This area of research is rapidly evolving. Current insights will likely be expanded significantly with a substantial ongoing interest in levosimendan, particularly for more at-risk populations. Numerous ongoing studies, as listed on clinicaltrials.gov, are actively recruiting patients for further investigation.

Does levosimendan improve renal outcomes in cardiac surgery patients?
Levosimendan's potential to enhance renal outcomes in cardiac surgery patients was explored in a recent study.[9] This drug increases renal blood flow through vasodilation, leading to a rise in intra-glomerular pressure and filtration. However, its direct impact on acute kidney injury (AKI) post-cardiac surgery had not been thoroughly investigated until this 2021 study.

In a single-center RCT, 29 patients who developed AKI within the first 48 hours following cardiac surgery were selected. These patients were hemodynamically stable and were randomized to receive either levosimendan or a placebo. The primary outcomes measured included renal blood flow and renal vascular resistance. Results demonstrated improvements in these parameters with the use of levosimendan.

An important observation was the augmentation of MAP to 70-80 mmHg, when necessary, using norepinephrine in both study groups. Notably, this intervention was more frequently required in the levosimendan group. Despite these findings, the study concluded that levosimendan did not significantly impact the glomerular filtration rate (GFR), a key measure of kidney function.

What about levosimendan in peripartum cardiomyopathy?
In a 2014 RCT, 30 patients with peripartum cardiomyopathy were administered levosimendan or milrinone.[10] Initially, these patients had a baseline cardiac index of 1.1-1.3 L/min/m². After 24 hours, while both drugs improved cardiac index and stroke volume (SV), milrinone was significantly more effective than levosimendan. For instance, milrinone increased the baseline cardiac index from 1.3 to 4.3 L/min/m², compared to levosimendan's increase from 1.1 to 2.4 L/min/m². Despite this disparity in cardiac improvement, no differences were noted in other hemodynamic parameters or patient prognosis between the two groups.

Is levosimendan contraindicated in renal dysfunction patients?
There has been concern about using levosimendan in patients with a GFR < 30 ml/min/1.73m², as its package insert advises against use in severe renal impairment.[11] However, a 2021 study by Chan *et al.* compared levosimendan and dobutamine in 426 patients with an estimated GFR ≤ 30.[12] Dobutamine's package

110

insert doesn't consider renal function.[13] Their analysis, including propensity matching, demonstrated no significant difference in all-cause mortality between patients with an eGFR < 30 or on dialysis receiving levosimendan versus dobutamine. These findings suggest that an eGFR < 30 may not be a contraindication for levosimendan.

How does levosimendan compare to dobutamine in cardiogenic shock or low cardiac output syndrome?

A 2020 Cochrane Systematic Review investigating the treatment of cardiogenic shock or low cardiac output syndrome revealed no significant difference between levosimendan and dobutamine regarding short-term and long-term all-cause mortality and MAP.[14] However, levosimendan demonstrated advantages over dobutamine in improving cardiac index and reducing pulmonary capillary wedge pressure.

What about levosimendan versus enoximone in acute myocardial infarction cardiogenic shock?

A 2008 study by Fuhrmann compared enoximone, a phosphodiesterase inhibitor, with levosimendan in treating post-acute myocardial infarction (AMI) cardiogenic shock.[15] Conducted as an RCT with 32 patients, it observed a trend toward better survival with levosimendan, although the results were not statistically significant.

Can levosimendan be utilized in patients with septic shock?

Levosimendan's role in treating septic shock patients, particularly those with sepsis-induced cardiomyopathy, is complex. The 2016 LeoPARDS trial, which included 515 septic shock patients, demonstrated unfavorable outcomes for levosimendan, with increased risks of supraventricular tachyarrhythmia and prolonged mechanical ventilation.[5] It is worth noting that the baseline median cardiac index was 2.7 L/min/m². These patients did not have sepsis-induced cardiomyopathy as a cardiac index less than or equal to 2.2 L/min/m².

Similarly, a 2017 meta-analysis of seven trials with 258 patients found no superiority of levosimendan over dobutamine in reducing mortality or other outcomes in septic shock.[16] Due to safety concerns, cost, and limited availability, the 2021 *Surviving Sepsis Campaign* Guidelines issued a weak recommendation against levosimendan in this context.[1]

Recent developments in 2023 suggest a potential shift in the use of levosimendan for septic shock. A single-blind RCT by Sun *et al.*, involving 28 patients, indicated the benefits of levosimendan over dobutamine, such as improved cardiac index, reduced myocardial injury, and shorter mechanical ventilation time.[4] This study notably differed from the LeoPARDS trial in that patients had a baseline cardiac index below 2 L/min/m².

However, caution is warranted in interpreting these results.[17] The study's single-blind design, where only patients and their families were blinded, not clinicians, could introduce bias. Additionally, the small sample size, a result of a three-year enrollment at a single center, limits the generalizability of the findings. It is also important to note that the center did not provide mechanical circulatory support for patients refractory to these treatments, although such escalation has been suggested in the literature.

What adverse events can we expect with levosimendan?
The adverse events associated with levosimendan primarily include hypotension, atrial fibrillation, tachycardia, hypokalemia, and headache.[18] Hypotension was observed in 36.2% of cases, which is a significant concern due to the medication's effect on SVR. Atrial fibrillation was also reported in 14.1% of patients treated with levosimendan. Additionally, tachycardia, hypokalemia, and headache were frequently documented, highlighting the need for careful monitoring and management of these potential side effects.[2,18]

FUN FACTS!
Half-Life: One hour.[11]
Other Names: *Simdax*.[11]
Dosing: Clinical trials, including a 2023 study by Welker, recommend administering levosimendan with a loading dose of 6-12 µg/kg over 10 minutes, followed by a maintenance infusion rate of 0.05-0.2 µg/kg/min for 24 hours.[2]
Bolus Dosing Frequency: In practice, bolus dosing of levosimendan is utilized in 7.5% of cases.[19]
Concomitant Use with Other Vasopressors/Inotropes: 76.6% of levosimendan patients are also on inotropes or vasopressors.[19]

Citations
eddyjoemd.com/levosimendan-citations

16: METHYLENE BLUE

Chances are, if you are considering administering methylene blue to your patient, they are really sick—exit the comfort zone. You have hit the end of the traditional path. There are two main clinical situations where, as a vasopressor, methylene blue is considered: cardiac surgery-related vasoplegia and septic shock.

What is the mechanism of action of methylene blue?
Methylene blue could assist in managing profound vasodilation observed in distributive shock conditions, such as septic shock and cardiac surgery-related vasoplegia. This vasodilation is often triggered by cytokines and endotoxins that stimulate the production of inducible nitric oxide synthase (iNOS).[53] iNOS, in turn, leads to the production of nitric oxide (NO), a potent vasodilator. When present in excess, NO contributes to the vasodilation and resulting distributive shock commonly observed in these patients.[2] The action of NO activates soluble guanylate cyclase (sGC),[1] which then facilitates the generation of cyclic guanosine monophosphate (cGMP), leading to vasodilation.[44] Methylene blue intervenes by inhibiting both iNOS and sGC, effectively reducing the excessive vasodilation. While there are various descriptions of these mechanisms in medical literature, a simplified understanding is that methylene blue suppresses these vasodilators rather than directly causing vasoconstriction.[3]

In terms of the MAP = CO x SVR equation, methylene blue aims to normalize the low systemic vascular resistance (SVR). The data regarding the effects of methylene blue on cardiac output (CO) are not entirely clear. Some studies have suggested increased CO attributed to improved left ventricular filling and function.[56] Other research indicates that NO produced by iNOS interferes with the heart's ability to utilize adenosine triphosphate (ATP),[34] potentially reducing inotropy and CO. The exact effects of methylene blue on CO remain an area of ongoing investigation.

What adverse effects should we consider before ordering methylene blue?
When it comes to administering methylene blue, we must be acutely aware of its potential adverse effects, some of which can lead to significant harm if the drug is incorrectly administered. One of methylene blue's immediate, though relatively benign, effects is its propensity to turn the urine blue for about three days[4] and possibly cause bluish skin discoloration.[5]

Serotonin Syndrome
The more serious concern lies in the risk of serotonin syndrome. This risk becomes particularly pertinent in the management of cardiac surgery-related vasoplegia, where patients might already be on a range of medications influencing serotonin levels. For instance, many patients on selective serotonin reuptake inhibitors (SSRI), serotonin and norepinephrine reuptake inhibitors

(SNRI), or cyclic antidepressants could be at heightened risk when methylene blue is added to their regimen. This concern is amplified when considering medications like fentanyl, commonly utilized for analgesia in post-cardiac surgery patients. Fentanyl is a direct serotonin receptor agonist, and its combination with methylene blue can precipitate serotonin syndrome.[6-8]

Other seldom utilized post-cardiac surgery medications, such as tramadol for pain and meperidine for shivering,[9] also impair serotonin reuptake and can contribute to serotonin syndrome when combined with methylene blue. This risk is further compounded with the use of 5-HT3 receptor antagonists, such as ondansetron and granisetron, for postoperative nausea and vomiting. Various case reports have documented serotonin syndrome with combinations including methylene blue, such as paroxetine with granisetron,[10] fentanyl with citalopram,[6] fentanyl with sertraline,[11,12] and sertraline with mirtazapine and fentanyl.[13]

Similar precautions apply in the management of septic shock, especially when considering the addition of linezolid, an antibiotic that inhibits serotonin metabolism by inhibiting monoamine oxidase.[23] This interaction necessitates reevaluating methylene blue use in patients on linezolid.

While the Hunter Serotonin Toxicity Criteria and treatment for serotonin syndrome are beyond this book's scope, the existing black-box warning for methylene blue concerning serotonin syndrome underscores the need for cautious use.[51] In cases where the risk of serotonin syndrome is high, considering other catecholamine-sparing options, such as angiotensin II or hydroxocobalamin, might be prudent.[13-15]

Interference with Oximetry
Another aspect to consider is the interference of methylene blue with oximetry. Patients receiving this drug could demonstrate a false decrease in oxygen saturation on pulse oximetry due to the dye's interference with light transmission.[31] Even arterial blood gas analysis may not provide accurate readings, as different co-oximetry devices use various wavelengths that could be affected by methylene blue.[17] It is worth checking if methylene blue affects the equipment at your institution.

Pulmonary Vasoconstriction and Hypoxia
Methylene blue's effect on pulmonary function should not be overlooked. Increases in pulmonary vascular resistance (PVR) were first noted in a small, six-patient study of septic shock patients in 1995[18] and reiterated in a ten-patient 1999 study.[1] These findings caution against its use in patients with acute respiratory distress syndrome (ARDS) or pulmonary hypertension. However, more recent data involving patients with ARDS did not find issues with gas exchange, suggesting that the effect on pulmonary function may vary.[5] Nonetheless, it might

114

be wise to avoid methylene blue in patients with pulmonary hypertension or significant right ventricular dysfunction for the time being.[19]

Hemolytic Anemia

Acute hemolytic anemia is another complication associated with methylene blue, particularly at doses over 7 mg/kg.[20] This risk is especially pronounced in patients with glucose-6-phosphate dehydrogenase (G6PD) deficiency, who cannot metabolize methylene blue effectively.[21-23] Therefore, caution is advised when considering methylene blue in G6PD deficient patients.

How do we dose methylene blue?

There are a range of practices mainly due to the variability in existing data when dosing methylene blue. Typically, doses range between 1 and 2 mg/kg.[24] This variation is evident in clinical trials, with the most common dosing being around 2 mg/kg.[25] In certain scenarios, like for patients on the cardio-pulmonary bypass circuit, a higher dose of 3 mg/kg has been utilized to account for the additional volume of the circuit.[26] However, determining the optimal dose for patients on extracorporeal membrane oxygenation (ECMO) remains challenging due to additional factors like tubing and the oxygenator.[24] The duration of infusion can also vary, ranging from 20 minutes to over an hour.[3] Some treatment protocols extend the infusion to a continuous 24-hour period following the initial bolus.[27] However, caution is advised with doses higher than 2 mg/kg, as they have been linked to detrimental effects, including cardiac arrhythmias, coronary vasoconstriction, decreased cardiac output, and mesenteric and renal blood flow.[31]

An interesting example of methylene blue dosing in clinical trials is the SHOCKEM-Blue trial, which investigated its use in septic shock patients.[5] In this study, 100 mg of methylene blue was diluted in a 500 mL 0.9% NaCl bag and infused over 6 hours daily for three days. This dosing regimen was chosen based on the prolonged inflammatory insult characteristic of septic shock, as opposed to the shorter duration typically observed in cardiac surgery-related vasoplegia. The fixed dosing was also a matter of convenience, aligning with the vial sizes available at the hospital and falling within the beneficial range indicated in other studies. Dosing schemes in clinical research can sometimes be arbitrary. The choice of regimen in the SHOCKEM-Blue trial reflects this, and it is crucial to recognize that if this specific regimen did not yield positive results, it should not wholly dismiss methylene blue's potential efficacy in septic shock. Future research is needed to uncover more about its optimal dosing, especially in different clinical contexts.

What is the half-life of methylene blue?

The half-life of methylene blue ranges from 5 to 6 hours.[3,29] Research indicates a significant decrease in plasma concentrations around 40 minutes following administration.[3] Conversely, other studies suggest that the peak pharmacological

115

response of methylene blue is observed approximately 2 hours after initiation.[30] These variations in pharmacokinetics underpin the rationale for considering a continuous infusion following an initial bolus dose.

Should we provide an infusion after the bolus dose of methylene blue?
The question of whether to follow up a bolus dose of methylene blue with a continuous infusion has garnered attention in clinical practice, especially given the variability in dosing strategies for this medication. Hohlfelder and colleagues conducted a retrospective analysis at the Cleveland Clinic to explore this issue.[28] They looked at patient outcomes in cases where only a bolus was given compared to those where a bolus was followed by a continuous infusion specifically in treating cardiac surgery-related vasoplegia. Interestingly, their findings in the small 44-patient sample size did not indicate a clear benefit from providing a continuous infusion of methylene blue after the initial bolus dose.

When was methylene blue first described in the cardiac surgery literature?
The first documented use of methylene blue in cardiac surgery-related vasoplegia dates back to 1999.[35] It is remarkable to consider that, despite over two decades of use in this field, the literature on methylene blue remains somewhat limited in scope. A significant contribution to this body of research is a systematic review and meta-analysis published in 2021. This analysis demonstrated that as an adjunct in the treatment of cardiac surgery-related vasoplegia, methylene blue significantly reduced the incidence of renal failure, multiple organ failure, and overall mortality.[36]

Will our patient respond to methylene blue?
It is essential to recognize that not every therapy is universally effective for every patient, and methylene blue is no exception. This point is particularly crucial as have observed clinicians discarding potentially beneficial treatments after a single unsuccessful attempt. In the case of methylene blue, specific research indicates a therapeutic response rate of approximately 44%.[30]

Understanding how 'response rate' is defined in this context is vital. In the cited study, a positive response was identified as a 20% reduction in the dosage of norepinephrine or vasopressin.[30] Interestingly, if the criteria for a positive response is adjusted to a 10% decrease in these vasopressor doses, the response rate to methylene blue increases to about 56%.[37] While these figures are significant, they are still far from a universal 100% success rate.

Should we provide prophylactic methylene blue before cardiac surgery?
Given that cardiac surgery-related vasoplegia affects 5-25% of cardiac surgery patients,[30] considering prophylactic administration of methylene blue in patients with risk factors is a logical step. This approach has been evaluated in two trials. In a 2005 study, 50 patients identified as at risk for vasoplegic syndrome due to their use of calcium channel blockers and angiotensin-converting enzyme (ACE

116

inhibitors were given 2 mg/kg of methylene blue one hour before cardiac surgery.[4] Compared to a placebo group, these patients exhibited a higher SVR, required fewer vasopressors, and experienced shorter ICU and hospital stays. Another 30-patient trial in 2006 focused on patients on ACE inhibitors, administering methylene blue (3 mg/kg) or a placebo at the onset of cardiopulmonary bypass.[26] The methylene blue group demonstrated increased MAP and SVR and a reduced need for vasopressors compared to the placebo group. These findings suggest that patients who received methylene blue prophylactically in the preoperative and intraoperative periods were less likely to develop cardiac surgery-related vasoplegia and had improved outcomes.

What about administering methylene blue in septic shock?
Methylene blue has been explored as a treatment for septic shock since 1995, with initial trials noting improvements in MAP and SVR.[18] Early randomized controlled trials (RCTs) in the 2000s, involving 20 and 30 patients, demonstrated improved vasopressor requirements and MAP, although these studies were not powered to assess other outcomes.[44,45] A subsequent systematic review and meta-analysis, incorporating various small randomized and non-randomized studies, indicated the potential benefits of methylene blue on MAP.[25] Reviews of case reports, non-randomized trials, and retrospective studies echoed these findings, demonstrating improvements in MAP, SVR, and reduced vasopressor requirements.[22]

The use of methylene blue in septic shock gained renewed interest with the 2023 SHOCKEM-Blue trial conducted by Ibarra-Estrada et al., an RCT involving 91 patients with septic shock.[5] The study's primary outcome was the time to vasopressor discontinuation, which demonstrated a significant reduction in the methylene blue group (median of 69 hours) compared to the control group (median of 94 hours). The secondary outcome of vasopressor-free days at 28 days also favored methylene blue.

The methylene blue group experienced a shorter shock duration and a significantly lower cumulative fluid balance, about 750 mL less than the control group. However, no differences were observed in mechanical ventilation and mortality days, though trends suggested potential improvements. The study also reported shorter ICU and hospital stays for patients receiving methylene blue, with median discharges occurring 1.5 and 2.7 days sooner, respectively.

Despite the lack of a statistically significant mortality benefit, several points merit discussion. The efforts of Ibarra-Estrada et al. in early patient identification and initiation of appropriate therapies, coupled with the use of evidence-based strategies for fluid responsiveness, are commendable. Yet, the mortality rate in the control group was notably high at 46%, surpassing rates observed in other septic shock trials like PROMISE, PROCESS, and ARISE.[46-48] This high mortality rate took place in patients with a higher APACHE score than the PROMISE trial, reflecting the real-world challenges in managing septic shock patients. The methylene blue group exhibited a 33% mortality rate at 28 days, which, while lower than the control group, was not statistically significant. Given these findings, more extensive studies are needed to conclusively determine methylene blue's impact on mortality and other vital outcomes in septic shock.

Are we ready for routine use of methylene blue in sepsis?
Currently, the available data do not robustly support the routine use of methylene blue for septic shock. However, there is potential for its earlier application in the future. As Teja et al. highlighted, the risk-benefit ratios of methylene blue in these contexts remain unclear.[49] Despite this, the landscape could shift, as indicated by a meta-analysis of randomized trials that reported reductions in mortality and decreases in ICU and hospital lengths of stay using methylene blue.[12]

Could ECMO patients benefit from methylene blue?
In a small retrospective study focusing on patients undergoing extracorporeal membrane oxygenation (ECMO; predominantly veno-arterial or VA ECMO), researchers investigated whether methylene blue could effectively improve blood pressure and potentially survival.[37] The study found that 55.6% of patients experienced an improvement in their MAP, with an increase of 10% or more occurring within 1 to 2 hours post-administration. Notably, all patients who did not achieve at least a 5% increase in MAP ultimately did not survive. While the study was not designed to assess survival benefits directly, it was observed that 32% of those who responded to methylene blue survived, compared to only 10% of non-responders.

Where else has methylene blue been utilized?
Methylene blue has found applications beyond its use in cardiac surgery and sepsis. Notably, patients undergoing liver transplantation often experience shock states due to postreperfusion syndrome and ischemia-reperfusion injury.[19,53] In these cases, methylene blue has been administered with varying results, which are beyond the detailed exploration of this book. Additionally, methylene blue has demonstrated promise as an adjunct therapy in anaphylaxis, with its efficacy documented in various case reports and case series.[19,20]

What's the next step for methylene blue?
The future of methylene blue in clinical practice should not be shrouded in decades of uncertainty. Teja et al. recommend reserving methylene blue for cases of shock refractory to multiple vasopressors and corticosteroids.[49] At present, its use in sepsis remains a subject of debate due to the limited evidence base.[50] Despite this, some clinicians advocate for its earlier deployment in sepsis management.[54] While the application of methylene blue in cardiac surgery-related vasoplegia is broadly accepted, its role in treating septic shock continues to be a topic of considerable debate.

FUN FACTS!

Early Experiments: Methylene blue's history in medical experimentation dates back to 1891 when Paul Erlich tested it in malaria patients.[55]

FDA Approval: Methylene blue was FDA-approved much later, in 2016.[51]

FDA-Approved Clinical Indication: The primary indication of methylene blue is in managing methemoglobinemia.[31,51] It facilitates the conversion of methemoglobin back to hemoglobin, an essential process for effectively transporting oxygen throughout the body.

Citations

eddyjoemd.com/methylene-blue-citations

17: HYDROXOCOBALAMIN

Hydroxocobalamin is a high-dose IV formulation of vitamin B12a that received FDA approval in 1975 for treating known or suspected cyanide poisoning.[1] Despite being one of the body's four forms of vitamin B12,[2] we may find it in the literature under multiple names, including hydroxocobalamin, vitamin B12, and vitamin B12a.[3] Remarkably, the use of hydroxocobalamin for distributive shock originated accidentally, with 18-28% of patients receiving it for cyanide toxicity experiencing an unexpected side effect: extreme hypertension.[4] This scenario is reminiscent of stories where some unintended consequences lead to a new medical invention, such as the discovery of *Viagra*. Like methylene blue, hydroxocobalamin was explored as a catecholamine-sparing agent in cardiac surgery-related vasoplegia and septic shock. Existing literature mainly comprises case reports, case series, and cohort studies. Thus, we only have one pilot trial on septic shock to glean insights from at the time of writing.[5]

What is the mechanism of action of hydroxocobalamin?
Much like methylene blue, hydroxocobalamin rids the body of vasodilator properties rather than causing direct vasoconstriction. Over the years, its exact mechanism of action has been refined through experimentation. The initial theories revolved around modifications to nitric oxide metabolism.[6] Like methylene blue, hydroxocobalamin inhibits nitric oxide synthase, which is upregulated by inflammatory cytokines and interleukins.[7] Nitric oxide synthase leads to the production of nitric oxide, a potent vasodilator. Moreover, hydroxocobalamin also directly inhibits nitric oxide.[2] Additionally, it hinders soluble guanylate cyclase (sGC), an enzyme that generates cyclic guanosine monophosphate (cGMP), another vasodilator.[2]

Beyond its impact on nitric oxide, hydroxocobalamin has another ace up its sleeve. It also inhibits hydrogen sulfide (H2S), which is another culprit of the vasodilation our patients experience.[6,9] The details of how H2S causes vasodilation are beyond the scope of this book, as current papers describe a "proposed mechanism of action" rather than providing definitive explanations.[10] The inhibition of H2S is a distinct aspect of hydroxocobalamin, differentiating it from methylene blue.

In the MAP = CO x SVR equation, hydroxocobalamin should increase systemic vascular resistance (SVR) due to its effect on NO and H2S. This would yield an increase in the mean arterial pressure (MAP). There is no reported direct effect on cardiac output (CO).

What adverse effects should we prepare for?

We live and die by lab values. Multi-system organ failure is expected when a patient is sufficiently ill for us to go down the hydroxocobalamin pathway. When a patient's condition is severe enough to warrant hydroxocobalamin, the preparation and understanding of potential adverse effects are essential.

Ensuring your colleagues and staff are well-informed regarding these lab value interferences is vital. For instance, we want to avoid making mistakes in patient management simply due to a spurious lab result. Thankfully, these interferences typically resolve within 48 hours.[12] Notably, the IV-HOCSS trial did not encounter lab issues in the ten patients who received hydroxocobalamin for septic shock.[5] Fortunately, it does not appear that the I-STAT measurements are impacted by hydroxocobalamin. However, it is crucial to assess how hydroxocobalamin may impact devices utilized in your institution.[12]

- **CBC with differential:** Prepare for elevated hemoglobin and basophil levels for 12 to 16 hours.[1,10] Lymphocytopenia could also occur.[11]
- **Chemistry:** Creatinine, glucose, albumin, total protein, and alkaline phosphatase may be elevated for up to 24 hours.[1] The renal function becomes tricky as hydroxocobalamin can cause acute kidney injury (AKI) due to oxalate nephropathy.[11,19] Oxalate crystals can be found in over 50% of patients, although the IV-HOCSS trial reported zero such incidences.[5] The interpretation of increased creatinine can be challenging, as it may be affected by underlying shock, oxalate nephropathy, or potentially falsely elevated values. We are left scratching our heads as medicine further becomes an art rather than a science. Bilirubin may be elevated in the liver function tests for four days. For patients on mechanical circulatory support, consider shifting from trending lactate dehydrogenase (LDH) to monitoring plasma-free hemoglobin,[10] as LDH can be unpredictable after hydroxocobalamin administration.
- **Coagulation Studies:** Be prepared for the unpredictability of PT/INR and PTT results for up to two days.[10]
- **Cosmetic findings:** Prepare for up to six weeks of red urine, as chromaturia occurs in all patients receiving hydroxocobalamin.[10]. Remember how described methylene blue, making urine blue in the previous chapter? I am curious whether the patients who received methylene blue and hydroxocobalamin in studies ended up with purple urine. I digress. Furthermore, expect erythema in 94% of patients due to inadequate medication absorption.[1] This erythema should not be confused with an allergy. Dermatology consults and corticosteroid prescriptions are not warranted. Some patients may also experience up to two weeks of photosensitivity and an acneiform rash, occurring in at least 20% of patients.[1,10]
- **Device malfunctions:** Patients on dialysis may encounter issues when receiving hydroxocobalamin. If blood leak alarms occur during dialysis, it is due to the medication's dark red color.[1,10,11,13] This alarm has been described in the Fresenius 2008K machine.[10] The alarm's duration can extend for over eight days, and there may also be complications with specific ECMO sensors.[10,]

Nephrologists and ECMO specialists should be consulted to address these potential malfunctions using hydroxocobalamin.

Can we use hydroxocobalamin for cardiac surgery-related vasoplegia?
Hydroxocobalamin was studied in a cohort of 198 patients with cardiac surgery-related vasoplegia.[14] In patients at risk of serotonin syndrome or with underlying G6PD deficiency, it serves as a backup option when methylene blue may be inappropriate.[4] The most extensive case series—involving 33 patients—demonstrated improvements in MAP and vasopressor requirements in approximately 73% of patients.[13] Furthermore, reviews of case reports and series repeatedly illustrate improved MAP and reduced vasopressor requirements.[14] It is imperative to acknowledge that these findings are subject to publication bias, as negative results are less likely to be reported by the authors.

What is the dose of hydroxocobalamin for cardiac surgery-related vasoplegia?
A systematic review and meta-analysis extracted the dosing schemes from multiple studies.[14] The most commonly utilized dosing regimen mirrors that used for cyanide poisoning, which is 5 g IV administered over 15 minutes.[1] A single dose is the most commonly used. However, it can be repeated.[11,14] The time intervals between the doses vary and necessitate further investigation. Using three doses was described once.[15]

When was hydroxocobalamin first utilized in septic shock?
The application of hydroxocobalamin in septic shock originates from its potential to influence the SVR component in the MAP = CO x SVR equation through its impact on nitric oxide and hydrogen sulfide. The first reported use of hydroxocobalamin for septic shock occurred in 2018 when two patients experienced increased MAP and reduced vasopressor requirements.[3] This report was followed by a case series involving 26 patients with similar results, including MAP improvement and reduced vasopressor requirements.[17]

IV-HOCSS: IV HydrOxoCobalamin in Septic Shock Trial
The IV-HOCSS trial, as a Phase II trial, was not designed nor powered to be revolutionary.[5] See 'The Basics' chapter for a breakdown of the different phases of clinical trials. The trial enrolled 20 septic shock patients who received fluids, cultures, antibiotics, and vasopressors within 24 hours of admission.[5] While this sample size is small, it is important to remember that the purpose was not to recruit a large number of patients but to assess the treatment's early efficacy. Right off the bat, we can throw mortality, length of stay, and such endpoints out the door, as these cannot be appropriately evaluated.

The study's primary outcome was feasibility, which it attained.[5] The secondary outcome focused on H2S level variations before and after infusion and norepinephrine dosage changes. Notably, the study revealed a statistically significant change in monobromobimane-reactive H2S levels and a reduction in norepinephrine dosage, suggesting a catecholamine-sparing effect. The investigators checked the H2S level before and half an hour after infusion. In addition, they noted the norepinephrine dose at randomization, one minute before the B12 was given, 30 minutes after, and three hours later. There was only a statistically significant difference in the one-minute to 30-minute window. Tertiary outcomes, such as mortality and length of stay, did not demonstrate significant differences, and no adverse effects were reported. While the lack of vital outcomes aligns with the expectations of a Phase II trial, further research is needed to justify routine hydroxocobalamin use due to its cost and limited data.

Is the dosing of hydroxocobalamin different in septic shock?
The IV-HOCSS trial also utilized 5 g IV.[5] This dose likely stems from the convenience of hydroxocobalamin already available in a 5 g form. Furthermore, data support the safety of this dose.

How long will the effects of hydroxocobalamin last?
A retrospective case series involving a cohort of 35 patients discovered that the hemodynamic benefits of hydroxocobalamin largely dissipated within 24 hours.[16] Only 17.1% of patients had a MAP increase of > 5 mHg at 24 hours. Unfortunately, the IV-HOCSS trial only monitored patients for up to three hours.[5]

What response rate can we expect?
It is vital to comprehend that hydroxocobalamin—like most other medical interventions—does not assure a 100% response rate. Past data indicates that approximately 27% of patients do not respond to hydroxocobalamin.[13]

What's the next step with hydroxocobalamin?
These data on hydroxocobalamin in cardiac surgery-related vasoplegia and septic shock provide a foundation for further trials investigating nitric oxide and H2S modulation in critically ill patients. However, enrolling patients in such studies may be challenging, as hydroxocobalamin is often considered a last-resort measure. Many questions remain regarding its effectiveness, patient selection criteria, timing of administration, and dosage.[18]

FUN FACTS!
FDA approval: 1975
How long has hydroxocobalamin been utilized elsewhere?
Hydroxocobalamin has been utilized for cyanide poisoning for over 50 years in Europe.[2]

Citations
eddyjoemd.com/hydroxocobalamin-citations

18: HYDROXOCOBALAMIN VS. METHYLENE BLUE

Head to Head: Which is Better?

Selecting an optimal rescue strategy in cardiac surgery-related vasoplegia, especially when other vasopressors are ineffective in elevating systemic vascular resistance (SVR), is challenging due to limited data. The question arises: should we opt for additional catecholamines, methylene blue, or hydroxocobalamin? Although direct comparative data for methylene blue and hydroxocobalamin in septic shock is absent, insights can be gleaned from retrospective studies in cardiac surgery-related vasoplegia.

A 2020 retrospective study by Furnish *et al.* involving 35 patients suggested that both methylene blue and hydroxocobalamin effectively increased mean arterial pressure (MAP) and SVR.[1] Another retrospective analysis at Duke involved 142 patients, but the distribution was uneven: only 22 received hydroxocobalamin compared to the rest receiving methylene blue.[2] This study did not find significant differences between the two treatments. Intriguingly, a 2023 systematic review and meta-analysis indicated a higher MAP in cardiac surgery-related vasoplegia patients treated with hydroxocobalamin than methylene blue.[3]

A comprehensive retrospective analysis compared vasopressor requirements and hemodynamic changes in patients treated with either methylene blue or hydroxocobalamin.[4] The sample included 77 patients on hydroxocobalamin and 43 on methylene blue. Notably, more patients in the methylene blue group were on renin-angiotensin system (RAS) inhibitors (21% versus 6.5%). The outcomes favored hydroxocobalamin, demonstrating a more significant increase in MAP and reduced vasopressor requirement. Given these findings, it is a preferable choice alongside hydroxocobalamin's easier dosing and lack of serotonin syndrome risk.

If methylene blue fails, can we try hydroxocobalamin?

As the response rate to methylene blue has been shown to range between 44 and 56%,[5,6] we should have a next step in mind for when it is not efficacious. The first case reports of hydroxocobalamin after methylene blue were published in 2016 and 2017. In these case reports, patients unresponsive to methylene blue were responsive to hydroxocobalamin.[7,8] If your team attempts this, please publish your data. I would love to review it for the next edition of this book.

Should we try monotherapy with methylene blue first or provide combination therapy?

The question of whether to start with methylene blue monotherapy or combination therapy with hydroxocobalamin remains open. A retrospective study of 20 patients compared the efficacy of methylene blue alone to its combination with hydroxocobalamin.[9] The combination therapy demonstrated vasopressor reductions at one-hour post-infusion and allowed for lower doses of methylene blue. However, this study's numerous limitations warrant caution in implementing this combined approach routinely. Hopefully, this will be prospectively evaluated soon.

Cost of Methylene Blue and Hydroxocobalamin

Limited data shows that the differences in outcomes between methylene blue and hydroxocobalamin may be negligible.[1,2] When developing protocols at our institutions, our pharmacy colleagues hold us accountable for staying within budgets. Methylene blue's average wholesale price is $247.90 for a 50mg vial. For a hypothetical 100kg patient requiring a 2 mg/kg dose, the cost would be approximately $991.60.[10] In contrast, a standard 5 g dose of hydroxocobalamin costs around $985.58.[11] Surprisingly, the cost difference is minimal for a 100kg patient. These figures are particularly relevant given the usual discrepancies between the standard 70kg patient and real-world patient weights, emphasizing the need for cost-effective clinical decision-making. Make the best decision for your patient.

Citations

eddyjoemd.com/hcb-vs-mb-citations/

19: PERIPHERAL VASOPRESSORS

We will begin our discussion of peripheral vasopressors with a quick anecdote from my research career. My first publication graced the pages of The Journal of Intensive Care Medicine in 2017.[1] A research project was a requirement to complete my Critical Care Medicine fellowship. Dr. Sudhir Datar—a neurointensivist and faculty member—invited me to collaborate with him on a project. Before this, I had no interest in clinical research. I have always been, and continue to be, a boots-on-the-ground physician. Dr. Datar proposed numerous ideas for clinical trials, hoping one would catch my attention. Finally, his proposition to explore peripheral vasopressors made the light bulb in my head flicker on. The opportunity to publish an article to check off the box to complete my fellowship and decrease patient morbidity? Sign me up!

To date, I have a love-hate relationship with central lines. When my Emergency Medicine colleagues call me for an ICU admission, I get warm fuzzies when there is a right internal jugular central venous catheter (CVC) on the chest x-ray. My initial thought is, 'Oh good, this means that I don't have to do it.' For those coming up in medicine, please let this be a warning that the allure of placing central lines eventually fades. Let me backtrack a bit to elaborate on my practice patterns.

In the Emergency Department (ED), when a critically ill patient requires admission to the ICU, I receive a secure message via a text-like app from the staff. This message typically contains the patient's name, medical record number, and a working diagnosis. I quickly review the patient's chart before speaking with the emergency medicine physician. The 30 seconds spent studying the chart provide valuable insights into why the patient necessitates an ICU bed. Through the electronic medical record (EMR), I can assess what interventions have been performed, review lab and imaging results, check the medications they are receiving, and evaluate their IV access.

Suppose the ED physician informs me that the patient receives norepinephrine at 5 µg/min through a peripheral IV (PIV), and the hemodynamic fluctuations have stabilized. I do not question the need for a central line in that case. Sometimes, we can get patients over the hump with vasopressors through a PIV. If the patient is unstable and central line placement is imminent, using vasopressors through a PIV can be a valuable interim solution until the line is placed. Studies have demonstrated that initiating vasopressors through a peripheral IV before central line placement can lead to faster achievement of hemodynamic targets.[2,3] In the ICU, a well-tucked-in patient is genuinely appreciated.

However, placing a central line involves a significant investment of time, energy, and resources. For instance, this includes the cost of the central line kit and all the necessary accessories for the procedure. In addition, the time clinicians spend placing the central line is mirrored by a similar time commitment from the bedside nurse, who is usually present to assist. Inserting a central line is a zero-sum game, where the setup and placement time affect the entire care team, the care of other patients, and other interventions.

Let us not forget the most crucial component in this scenario: the patient. Informing a patient that a large needle and catheter will be inserted into their neck, groin, or chest understandably raises significant concern. Some patients even require pre-medication to manage their anxiety. In my practice, I am generous with lidocaine to ensure their comfort.

How often do we observe complications with central venous catheters?
Despite advancements over the decades aimed at reducing complications related to CVCs, they still occur. Older data illustrated that up to 15% of patients had CVC-related complications.[4] These complications included mechanical issues such as arterial injuries, hematomas, and pneumothorax in up to 19% of patients. Infectious complications were observed in up to 26% of patients, while thrombotic complications occurred in up to 26% of cases.

Thanks to quality improvement initiatives like chlorhexidine patches, DVT prophylaxis, and the use of ultrasound, significant progress has been made in minimizing the rates of CVC-associated complications. However, there is always some level of risk involved. The 3SITES trial, published in 2015, randomized patients to receive a CVC through an internal jugular (IJ), subclavian, or femoral vein.[5] The incidence of pneumothorax requiring a chest tube in subclavian CVCs was 1.5%. Fewer than 1.5% of patients developed symptomatic DVTs or bloodstream infections.

In 2021, a systematic review and meta-analysis examined the literature on peripheral vasopressors, including over 16,000 patients from 23 studies.[6] While data limitations — including only two randomized controlled trials (RCTs) — should be acknowledged, the authors concluded that the incidence of adverse events related to peripheral vasopressors was low, at just 1.8%. The optimal vasopressor concentrations and infusion duration remain debatable, as 14,385 of the 16,055 patients came from an operating room setting. It may not be a direct apples-to-apples comparison, but the 3SITES trial reported an adverse event rate of approximately 1.5%. Consequently, a difference between 1.8% and 1.5% does not warrant the continued mandatory CVC placement.

When should we opt for peripheral vasopressors?
Hemodynamic management of septic shock involves administering IV fluids followed by vasopressors if specific targets are not met. The updated 202

Surviving Sepsis Campaign Guidelines now recommend considering peripheral vasopressors rather than waiting for a CVC placement.[7] Even before these guidelines were updated, two studies had demonstrated benefits in initiating vasopressors earlier during the resuscitation of patients in septic shock.[2,3] The CENSER trial, for example, provided norepinephrine at a median of 93 minutes from the patient's arrival in the ED versus 193 minutes in the control group.[2] Fewer than 50% of patients had a CVC when starting norepinephrine. Patients receiving early norepinephrine attained improved shock control at six hours. They experienced less cardiogenic pulmonary edema and fewer new-onset arrhythmias among the adverse events.

A prospectively collected database study providing 'very-early vasopressors' (VE-VP) frequently utilized vasopressors through a PIV.[3] VE-VP was defined as vasopressors initiated before the first fluid load or within the next hour. VE-VP patients received fewer IV fluids and experienced other beneficial outcomes, such as increased mechanical ventilation-free days and lower 28-day mortality rates. These beneficial findings should be further explored in prospective studies. In other words, placing the order to administer norepinephrine through a PIV may be beneficial sooner than our current practice patterns allow.

In my practice, I maintain a low threshold for initiating vasopressors if fluid resuscitation does not achieve the desired effects. The sooner we start, the better, as long as the patient receives optimal resuscitation. Meeting the MAP target with vasopressors does not signal an end to our assessment for fluid responsiveness.

Where should we place the PIV to minimize complications?
Determining the optimal location for the PIV is crucial to reduce the complication rates. Garcia-Cardenas *et al.* have set criteria that could be adopted in hospital policies to optimize patient safety.[8] These criteria include placing the PIV when the vein diameter exceeds 4 mm, ensuring the upper extremity is contralateral to the blood pressure cuff, using an 18 or 20-gauge IV, and avoiding placement in the hand, wrist, or antecubital fossa. Blood should also return from the PIV site before initiating the vasopressor. The staff should assess the PIV's function every two hours to ensure its adequate function.

According to a systematic review and meta-analysis by Owen *et al.*, extravasation occurred in 3.05% of patients when the PIV was placed in the hand, compared to 1.19% when placed proximal to the wrist.[6] The *Surviving Sepsis Campaign* recommends placing the peripheral IV in a vein in or proximal to the antecubital fossa.[7] This recommendation is supported by the fact that 85% of extravasation injuries occurred distal to the antecubital or popliteal fossa.[9]

How long can we safely infuse vasopressors through a PIV?
Cardenas-Garcia and colleagues reported a mean duration of 49 ± 22 hours via a PIV, with a maximum duration of 72 hours.[8] Datar *et al.* reported a mean duration of 19 hours due to the specific patient population in their study.[1] They reported that 17% of patients received phenylephrine for up to 48 hours. Furthermore, a 2020 systematic review found a mean infusion duration of 22 hours.[10] A systematic review of extravasation injuries from PIVs reported local tissue injuries with a median infusion duration of 56 hours.[9]

These data illustrate that infusions greater than 24 hours are generally safe, but beyond 48 hours, the risk may increase and should be evaluated case-by-case. A PICC line could become necessary. In my practice, when peripheral vasopressors are administered, we reassess the need for a CVC at least daily.

How high can we go with the doses of vasopressors?
When dosing norepinephrine and phenylephrine through a PIV, we primarily have retrospective studies to guide us. Data for dopamine, vasopressin, and epinephrine are available, but the sample sizes are small. It is worth noting that it is unknown whether one vasopressor is safer than another in case of extravasation. Let us break down the dosing for each vasopressor and provide insights from various studies:

Norepinephrine:
• Lewis *et al.*: Median: 0.08 µg/kg/min, Max: 0.13 µg/kg/min.[11]
• Cardenas-Garcia *et al.*: Mean: 0.70 ± 0.23 µg/kg/min.[8]
• Medjel *et al.*: Max 30 µg/min.[12]
Phenylephrine:
• Cardenas-Garcia *et al.*: Mean: 3.25 ± 1.69 µg/kg/min.[8]
• Datar *et al.*: Mean: 1.04 µg/kg/min, Max: 3.49 µg/kg/min.[1]
• Lewis *et al.*: Median: 50 µg/min, Max 95 µg/min.[11]
• Delgado *et al.*: Max 2 µg/kg/min.[13]

How do we classify extravasation injuries?
Two grading systems are available to help us define the extent and management of extravasation injuries: one developed by the U.S. Department of Health and Human Services/National Institute of Health (NIH) and another by the Society of Infusion Nursing.[14,15] Defining extravasation injuries can become challenging, as these classification systems are not consistently described in the literature.

The NIH Grading Scale defines Grade 1 as no big deal with painless edema, and the skin is intact.[14] Grade 2 is when we observe blanching of the skin or erythema. In the case of Grade 3, things get scary, and surgical evaluation is required for severe tissue damage. From here on, we start to observe tissue necrosis or ulceration. I cannot say I have ever witnessed a Grade 4 or 5 with life-threatening consequences or death, respectively.

The Society of Infusion Nursing provides more detail about the lesions but no therapeutic considerations compared to the NIH grading scale.[15] In Grade 0, the patient has no symptoms. Grades 1 and 2 have blanching of the skin. The difference is that in Grade 1, the edema is less than one inch versus one to six inches in Grade 2. These are cool, and pain could be present or absent. Grade 3 has edema greater than six inches but is accompanied by mild to moderate pain with some possible numbness. Grade 4 is accompanied by moderate to severe pain. Here, we may observe skin discoloration, bruising, and significant edema over six inches. Tight, leaking skin with pitting edema is also present.

How concerned should we be about extravasation injuries?
Cardenas-Garcia et al. reported extravasation injuries in 2% of patients.[8] Datar et al. observed a rate of 3%.[1] Furthermore, Medlej et al. found that 5.5% of their patients had extravasations, but fortunately, none required any treatment.[12] In another study by Lewis et al., 4% of patients experienced extravasations, with none requiring interventions.[11]

The most extensive retrospective cohort study involved 14,385 patients receiving anesthesia for surgical procedures.[16] This study reported only five cases of norepinephrine extravasation, which amounts to just 0.035% of the patients. None of these patients required any treatment. It is worth noting that the relatively short duration of the surgical cases played a role, making it an outlier compared to other clinical scenarios.

Should we worry about the norepinephrine concentration?
It would be prudent to consider using lower-concentration formulations of norepinephrine to minimize potential damage in case of extravasation. Our pharmacist colleagues can assist with the concentrations.

How should we manage extravasation injuries?
In the event of extravasation, our nurse colleagues should promptly notify the medical team and automatically initiate treatment. The package insert for norepinephrine recommends treating extravasation ischemia with 5 - 10 mg of phentolamine, an adrenergic-blocking agent, dissolved in 10 to 15 cc of saline solution.[17] A fine, hypodermic needle should be utilized to infiltrate the area liberally.

I prefer the guidance provided by Garcia-Cardenas et al., which involves several steps.[8] First, stop the vasopressor infusion. Aspirate any residual medication from the PIV site and remove the catheter. Outline the cutaneous lesion to establish a baseline for assessing the extent. Reconstitute the phentolamine and inject 0.5 to 1.0 cc in five different sites around the lesion's edges using a different 25 or 27-gauge needle for each injection. In addition, apply nitroglycerin paste to the area of extravasation.

Where to next?

If your institution lacks policies and procedures for using peripheral vasopressors, I recommend creating them. While there may be a lack of RCTs that we desire, the available data is sufficient to establish the safety of peripheral vasopressors. Enrolling critically ill patients in an RCT comparing peripheral IV to central venous catheter (CVC) usage for shock is challenging. Explaining to a patient with septic shock that they could either receive the vasopressor via a PIV in their arm or have a large catheter inserted in their neck is not a decision made lightly.

Therefore, when I order peripheral vasopressors for my patients, I ensure they (or their loved ones) comprehend the current situation and why we are initiating them. Furthermore, I always discuss the associated risks and obtain consent for a CVC should it become necessary.

Citations

eddyjoemd.com/peripheral-vasopressors-citations/

20: CONCLUSIONS

As we wrap up this book, it is evident that managing critically ill patients is a complex and evolving field. Throughout this book, we have delved into the pharmacological nuances, clinical applications, and evidence-based practices surrounding these vasopressors and inotropes. I have also told some lame jokes and anecdotes along the way.

One of the key themes that repeatedly emerged is the importance of individualized patient care. Each patient presents unique challenges, necessitating a tailored approach to vasopressor and inotrope therapy. This book has emphasized the critical role of continuous monitoring and adjustment of treatment based on the patient's hemodynamics. Not every patient reads the textbook.

In the ever-evolving landscape of critical care medicine, ongoing research and clinical trials continue to refine our understanding and use of these drugs. As such, this handbook serves as a foundation, a starting point for continued learning and adaptation in the face of new evidence and clinical experiences. I have learned a lot in writing this, and hopefully, you have picked up a thing or two along the way.

Thank you for choosing this book. Your support is invaluable, and I sincerely hope you find it a worthwhile investment. This project has been a passionate endeavor for me, filled with valuable learning experiences.

Your encouragement has been a significant motivator throughout this journey. For those discovering my work for the first time through this book, I invite you to explore my extensive array of free content. Please visit my website, eddyjoemd.com, and connect with me on social media platforms like Instagram, Facebook, X, and YouTube under the handle @eddyjoemd, as well as listen to The Saving Lives Podcast. Your engagement and feedback are greatly appreciated.

- Eddy J. Gutierrez

CITATIONS

THE BASICS CITATIONS

1. DeMers D, Wachs D. Physiology, Mean Arterial Pressure. [Updated 2023 Apr 10]. In: StatPearls [Internet]. Treasure Island (FL): StatPearls Publishing; 2023 Jan-. Available from: https://www.ncbi.nlm.nih.gov/books/NBK538226/
2. Nasim Naderi, Chapter 11 - Hemodynamic Study, Editor(s): Majid Maleki, Azin Alizadehasl, Majid Haghjoo, Practical Cardiology (Second Edition), Elsevier, 2022, Pages 201-216, ISBN 9780323809153, https://doi.org/10.1016/B978-0-323-80915-3.00013-2 (https://www.sciencedirect.com/science/article/pii/B9780323809153000132)
3. Kiers HD, Hofstra JM, Wetzels JF. Oscillometric blood pressure measurements: differences between measured and calculated mean arterial pressure. Neth J Med. 2008 Dec;66(11):474-9. PMID: 19075313.
4. Kaufmann T, Cox EGM, Wiersema R, Hiemstra B, Eck RJ, Koster G, Scheeren TWL, Keus F, Saugel B, van der Horst ICC; SICS Study Group. Non-invasive oscillometric versus invasive arterial blood pressure measurements in critically ill patients: A post hoc analysis of a prospective observational study. J Crit Care. 2020 Jun;57:118-123. doi: 10.1016/j.jcrc.2020.02.013. Epub 2020 Feb 22. PMID: 32109843.
5. Smulyan H, Safar ME. Blood pressure measurement: retrospective and prospective views. Am J Hypertens. 2011 Jun;24(6):628-34. doi: 10.1038/ajh.2011.22. Epub 2011 Feb 24. PMID: 21350431.
6. Evans L, Rhodes A, Alhazzani W, Antonelli M, Coopersmith CM, French C, Machado FR, Mcintyre L, Ostermann M, Prescott HC, Schorr C, Simpson S, Wiersinga WJ, Alshamsi F, Angus DC, Arabi Y, Azevedo L, Beale R, Beilman G, Belley-Cote E, Burry L, Cecconi M, Centofanti J, Coz Yataco A, De Waele J, Dellinger RP, Doi K, Du B, Estenssoro E, Ferrer R, Gomersall C, Hodgson C, Møller MH, Iwashyna T, Jacob S, Kleinpell R, Klompas M, Koh Y, Kumar A, Kwizera A, Lobo S, Masur H, McGloughlin S, Mehta S, Mehta Y, Mer M, Nunnally M, Oczkowski S, Osborn T, Papathanassoglou E, Perner A, Puskarich M, Roberts J, Schweickert W, Seckel M, Sevransky J, Sprung CL, Welte T, Zimmerman J, Levy M. Surviving sepsis campaign: international guidelines for management of sepsis and septic shock 2021. Intensive Care Med. 2021 Nov;47(11):1181-1247. doi: 10.1007/s00134-021-06506-y. Epub 2021 Oct 2. PMID: 34599691; PMCID: PMC8486643.
7. Bruss ZS, Raja A. Physiology, Stroke Volume. [Updated 2022 Sep 12]. In: StatPearls [Internet]. Treasure Island (FL): StatPearls Publishing; 2023 Jan-. Available from: https://www.ncbi.nlm.nih.gov/books/NBK547686/
8. Lang RM, Borow KM, Neumann A, Janzen D. Systemic vascular resistance: an unreliable index of left ventricular afterload. Circulation. 1986 Nov;74(5):1114-23. doi: 10.1161/01.cir.74.5.1114. PMID: 3769169.
9. Marik PE, Baram M, Vahid B. Does central venous pressure predict fluid responsiveness? A systematic review of the literature and the tale of seven mares. Chest. 2008 Jul;134(1):172-8. doi: 10.1378/chest.07-2331. PMID: 18628220.
10. Marik PE. Iatrogenic salt water drowning and the hazards of a high central venous pressure. Ann Intensive Care. 2014 Jun 21;4:21. doi: 10.1186/s13613-014-0021-0. PMID: 25110606; PMCID: PMC4122823.
11. VanValkinburgh D, Kerndt CC, Hashmi MF. Inotropes and Vasopressors. [Updated 2023 Feb 19]. In: StatPearls [Internet]. Treasure Island (FL): StatPearls Publishing; 2023 Jan-. Available from: https://www.ncbi.nlm.nih.gov/books/NBK482411/
12. van Diepen S, Katz JN, Albert NM, Henry TD, Jacobs AK, Kapur NK, Kilic A, Menon V, Ohman EM, Sweitzer NK, Thiele H, Washam JB, Cohen MG; American Heart Association Council on Clinical Cardiology; Council on Cardiovascular and Stroke Nursing; Council on Quality of Care and Outcomes Research; and Mission: Lifeline. Contemporary Management of Cardiogenic Shock: A Scientific Statement From the American Heart Association. Circulation. 2017 Oct 17;136(16):e232-e268. doi: 10.1161/CIR.0000000000000525. Epub 2017 Sep 18. PMID: 28923988.
13. Jensen BC, O'Connell TD, Simpson PC. Alpha-1-adrenergic receptors: targets for agonist drugs to treat heart failure. J Mol Cell Cardiol. 2011 Oct;51(4):518-28. doi: 10.1016/j.yjmcc.2010.11.014. Epub 2010 Nov 28. PMID: 21118696; PMCID: PMC3085055.
14. Demiselle J, Fage N, Radermacher P, Asfar P. Vasopressin and its analogues in shock states: a review. Ann Intensive Care. 2020 Jan 22;10(1):9. doi: 10.1186/s13613-020-0628-2. PMID: 31970567; PMCID: PMC6975768.
15. Sparapani S, Millet-Boureima C, Oliver J, Mu K, Hadavi P, Kalostian T, Ali N, Avelar CM, Bardies M, Barrow B, Benedikt M, Biancardi G, Bindra R, Bui L, Chihab Z, Cossitt A, Costa J, Daigneault T, Dault J, Davidson I, Dias J, Dufour E, El-Khoury S, Farhangdoost N, Forget A, Fox A, Gebrael M, Gentile MC, Geraci O, Gnanapragasam A, Gomah E, Haber E, Hamel C, Iyanker T, Kalantzis C, Kamali S, Kassardjian E, Kontos HK, Le TBU, LoScerbo D, Low YF, Mac Rae D, Maurer F, Mazhar S, Nguyen A, Nguyen-Duong K, Osborne-Laroche C, Park HW, Parolin E, Paul-Cole K, Peer LS, Philippon M, Plaisir CA, Porras Marroquin J, Prasad S, Ramsarun R, Razzaq S, Rhainds S, Robin D, Scartozzi R, Singh D, Fard SS, Soroko M, Soroori Motlagh N, Stern K, Toro L, Toure MW, Tran-Huynh S, Trépanier-Chicoine S, Waddingham C, Weekes AJ, Wisniewski A, Gamberi C. The Biology of Vasopressin. Biomedicines. 2021 Jan 18;9(1):89. doi: 10.3390/biomedicines9010089. PMID: 33477721; PMCID: PMC7832310.
16. Kaufmann JE, Oksche A, Wollheim CB, Günther G, Rosenthal W, Vischer UM. Vasopressin-induced von Willebrand factor secretion from endothelial cells involves V2 receptors and cAMP. J Clin Invest. 2000 Jul;106(1):107-16. doi: 10.1172/JCI9516. PMID: 10880054; PMCID: PMC314363.
17. Busse LW, Barker N, Petersen C. Vasoplegic syndrome following cardiothoracic surgery-review of pathophysiology and update of treatment options. Crit Care. 2020 Feb 4;24(1):36. doi: 10.1186/s13054-020-2743-8. PMID: 32019600; PMCID: PMC7001322.
18. Argenziano M, Chen JM, Choudhri AF, Cullinane S, Garfein E, Weinberg AD, Smith CR Jr, Rose EA, Landry DW, Oz MC. Management of vasodilatory shock after cardiac surgery: identification of predisposing factors and use of a

novel pressor agent. J Thorac Cardiovasc Surg. 1998 Dec;116(6):973-80. doi: 10.1016/S0022-5223(98)70049-2. PMID: 9832689.
19. Mazzeffi M, Hammer B, Chen E, Caridi-Scheible M, Ramsay J, Paciullo C. Methylene blue for postcardiopulmonary bypass vasoplegic syndrome: A cohort study. Ann Card Anaesth. 2017 Apr-Jun;20(2):178-181. doi: 10.4103/aca.ACA_237_16. PMID: 28393777; PMCID: PMC5408522.
20. Khanna A, English SW, Wang XS, Ham K, Tumlin J, Szerlip H, Busse LW, Altaweel L, Albertson TE, Mackey C, McCurdy MT, Boldt DW, Chock S, Young PJ, Krell K, Wunderink RG, Ostermann M, Murugan R, Gong MN, Panwar R, Hästbacka J, Favory R, Venkatesh B, Thompson BT, Bellomo R, Jensen J, Kroll S, Chawla LS, Tidmarsh GF, Deane AM; ATHOS-3 Investigators. Angiotensin II for the Treatment of Vasodilatory Shock. N Engl J Med. 2017 Aug 3;377(5):419-430. doi: 10.1056/NEJMoa1704154. Epub 2017 May 21. PMID: 28528561.
21. Beaulieu JM, Espinoza S, Gainetdinov RR. Dopamine receptors - IUPHAR Review 13. Br J Pharmacol. 2015 Jan;172(1):1-23. doi: 10.1111/bph.12906. PMID: 25671228; PMCID: PMC4280963.
22. Russell JA, Gordon AC, Williams MD, Boyd JH, Walley KR, Kissoon N. Vasopressor Therapy in the Intensive Care Unit. Semin Respir Crit Care Med. 2021 Feb;42(1):59-77. doi: 10.1055/s-0040-1710320. Epub 2020 Aug 20. PMID: 32820475.
23. Marik PE. Low-dose dopamine: a systematic review. Intensive Care Med. 2002 Jul;28(7):877-83. doi: 10.1007/s00134-002-1346-y. Epub 2002 May 31. PMID: 12122525.
24. Beck GCh, Brinkkoetter P, Hanusch C, Schulte J, van Ackern K, van der Woude FJ, Yard BA. Clinical review: immunomodulatory effects of dopamine in general inflammation. Crit Care. 2004 Dec;8(6):485-91. doi: 10.1186/cc2879. Epub 2004 Jun 3. PMID: 15566620; PMCID: PMC1065039.
25. Hasegawa D, Ishisaka Y, Maeda T, Prasitlumkum N, Nishida K, Dugar S, Sato R. Prevalence and Prognosis of Sepsis-Induced Cardiomyopathy: A Systematic Review and Meta-Analysis. J Intensive Care Med. 2023 Jun 4:8850666231180526. doi: 10.1177/08850666231180526. Epub ahead of print. PMID: 37272081.

NOREPINEPHRINE CITATIONS

1. Scheeren TWL, Bakker J, De Backer D, Annane D, Asfar P, Boerma EC, Cecconi M, Dubin A, Dünser MW, Duranteau J, Gordon AC, Hamzaoui O, Hernández G, Leone M, Levy B, Martin C, Mebazaa A, Monnet X, Morelli A, Payen D, Pearse R, Pinsky MR, Radermacher P, Reuter D, Saugel B, Sakr Y, Singer M, Squara P, Vieillard-Baron A, Vignon P, Vistisen ST, van der Horst ICC, Vincent JL, Teboul JL. Current use of vasopressors in septic shock. Ann Intensive Care. 2019 Jan 30;9(1):20. doi: 10.1186/s13613-019-0498-7. PMID: 30701448; PMCID: PMC6353977.
2. Evans L, Rhodes A, Alhazzani W, Antonelli M, Coopersmith CM, French C, Machado FR, Mcintyre L, Ostermann M, Prescott HC, Schorr C, Simpson S, Wiersinga WJ, Alshamsi F, Angus DC, Arabi Y, Azevedo L, Beale R, Beilman G, Belley-Cote E, Burry L, Cecconi M, Centofanti J, Coz Yataco A, De Waele J, Dellinger RP, Doi K, Du B, Estenssoro E, Ferrer R, Gomersall C, Hodgson C, Møller MH, Iwashyna T, Jacob S, Kleinpell R, Klompas M, Koh Y, Kumar A, Kwizera A, Lobo S, Masur H, McGloughlin S, Mehta S, Mehta Y, Mer M, Nunnally M, Oczkowski S, Osborn T, Papathanassoglou E, Perner A, Puskarich M, Roberts J, Schweickert W, Seckel M, Sevransky J, Sprung CL, Welte T, Zimmerman J, Levy M. Surviving sepsis campaign: international guidelines for management of sepsis and septic shock 2021. Intensive Care Med. 2021 Nov;47(11):1181-1247. doi: 10.1007/s00134-021-06506-y. Epub 2021 Oct 2. PMID: 34599691; PMCID: PMC8486643.
3. Giovannitti JA Jr, Thoms SM, Crawford JJ. Alpha-2 adrenergic receptor agonists: a review of current clinical applications. Anesth Prog. 2015 Spring;62(1):31-9. doi: 10.2344/0003-3006-62.1.31. PMID: 25849473; PMCID: PMC4389556.
4. Grignola JC, Domingo E. Acute Right Ventricular Dysfunction in Intensive Care Unit. Biomed Res Int. 2017;2017:8217105. doi: 10.1155/2017/8217105. Epub 2017 Oct 19. PMID: 29201914; PMCID: PMC5671685.
5. Levy B, Clere-Jehl R, Legras A, Morichau-Beauchant T, Leone M, Frederique G, Quenot JP, Kimmoun A, Cariou A, Lassus J, Harjola VP, Meziani F, Louis G, Rossignol P, Duarte K, Girerd N, Mebazaa A, Vignon P; Collaborators. Epinephrine Versus Norepinephrine for Cardiogenic Shock After Acute Myocardial Infarction. J Am Coll Cardiol. 2018 Jul 10;72(2):173-182. doi: 10.1016/j.jacc.2018.04.051. PMID: 29976201.
6. Morelli A, Ertmer C, Rehberg S, Lange M, Orecchioni A, Laderchi A, Bachetoni A, D'Alessandro M, Van Aken H, Pietropaoli P, Westphal M. Phenylephrine versus norepinephrine for initial hemodynamic support of patients with septic shock: a randomized, controlled trial. Crit Care. 2008;12(6):R143. doi: 10.1186/cc7121. Epub 2008 Nov 18. PMID: 19017409; PMCID: PMC2646303.
7. Dünser MW, Hasibeder WR. Sympathetic overstimulation during critical illness: adverse effects of adrenergic stress. J Intensive Care Med. 2009 Sep-Oct;24(5):293-316. doi: 10.1177/0885066609340519. Epub 2009 Aug 23. Erratum in: J Intensive Care Med. 2016 Sep;31(8):NP1. PMID: 19703817.
8. Jentzer JC, Coons JC, Link CB, Schmidhofer M. Pharmacotherapy update on the use of vasopressors and inotropes in the intensive care unit. J Cardiovasc Pharmacol Ther. 2015 May;20(3):249-60. doi: 10.1177/1074248414559838. Epub 2014 Nov 28. PMID: 25432872.
9. Russell JA, Gordon AC, Williams MD, Boyd JH, Walley KR, Kissoon N. Vasopressor Therapy in the Intensive Care Unit. Semin Respir Crit Care Med. 2021 Feb;42(1):59-77. doi: 10.1055/s-0040-1710320. Epub 2020 Aug 20. PMID: 32820475.
10. Bangash MN, Kong ML, Pearse RM. Use of inotropes and vasopressor agents in critically ill patients. Br J Pharmacol. 2012 Apr;165(7):2015-33. doi: 10.1111/j.1476-5381.2011.01588.x. PMID: 21740415; PMCID: PMC3413841.
11. Rokyta R Jr, Tesařová J, Pechman V, Gajdos P, Krouzecký A. The effects of short-term norepinephrine up-titration on hemodynamics in cardiogenic shock. Physiol Res. 2010;59(3):373-378. doi: 10.33549/physiolres.931804. Epub 2009 Aug 12. PMID: 19681659.

12. Thooft A, Favory R, Salgado DR, Taccone FS, Donadello K, De Backer D, Creteur J, Vincent JL. Effects of changes in arterial pressure on organ perfusion during septic shock. Crit Care. 2011;15(5):R222. doi: 10.1186/cc10462. Epub 2011 Sep 21. PMID: 21936903; PMCID: PMC3334768.
13. Hamzaoui O, Georger JF, Monnet X, Ksouri H, Maizel J, Richard C, Teboul JL. Early administration of norepinephrine increases cardiac preload and cardiac output in septic patients with life-threatening hypotension. Crit Care. 2010;14(4):R142. doi: 10.1186/cc9207. Epub 2010 Jul 29. PMID: 20670424; PMCID: PMC2945123.
14. Monnet X, Jabot J, Maizel J, Richard C, Teboul JL. Norepinephrine increases cardiac preload and reduces preload dependency assessed by passive leg raising in septic shock patients. Crit Care Med. 2011 Apr;39(4):689-94. doi: 10.1097/CCM.0b013e318206d2a3. PMID: 21263328.
15. LEVOPHED package insert, Lake Forest, IL: Hospira, Inc.; 2020.
16. "Vasopressin Injection, USP." FDA.gov, U.S. Food and Drug Administration, 2023.
17. Stefanou C, Palazis L, Loizou A, Timiliotou C. Should the norepinephrine maximal dosage rate be greatly increased in late shock? BMJ Case Rep. 2016 Mar 4;2016:bcr2015213670. doi: 10.1136/bcr-2015-213670. PMID: 26944371; PMCID: PMC4785500.
18. Brown SM, Lanspa MJ, Jones JP, Kuttler KG, Li Y, Carlson R, Miller RR 3rd, Hirshberg EL, Grissom CK, Morris AH. Survival after shock requiring high-dose vasopressor therapy. Chest. 2013 Mar;143(3):664-671. doi: 10.1378/chest.12-1106. PMID: 22911566; PMCID: PMC3590882.
19. Martin C, Medam S, Antonini F, Alingrin J, Haddam M, Hammad E, Meyssignac B, Vigne C, Zieleskiewicz L, Leone M. NOREPINEPHRINE: NOT TOO MUCH, TOO LONG. Shock. 2015 Oct;44(4):305-9. doi: 10.1097/SHK.0000000000000426. PMID: 26125087.
20. Auchet T, Regnier MA, Girerd N, Levy B. Outcome of patients with septic shock and high-dose vasopressor therapy. Ann Intensive Care. 2017 Dec;7(1):43. doi: 10.1186/s13613-017-0261-x. Epub 2017 Apr 20. PMID: 28425079; PMCID: PMC5397393.
21. Kasugai D, Hirakawa A, Ozaki M, Nishida K, Ikeda T, Takahashi K, Matsui S, Uenishi N. Maximum Norepinephrine Dosage Within 24 Hours as an Indicator of Refractory Septic Shock: A Retrospective Study. J Intensive Care Med. 2020 Nov;35(11):1285-1289. doi: 10.1177/0885066619860736. Epub 2019 Jun 27. PMID: 31248320.
22. Mouncey PR, Osborn TM, Power GS, Harrison DA, Sadique MZ, Grieve RD, Jahan R, Harvey SE, Bell D, Bion JF, Coats TJ, Singer M, Young JD, Rowan KM; ProMISe Trial Investigators. Trial of early, goal-directed resuscitation for septic shock. N Engl J Med. 2015 Apr 2;372(14):1301-11. doi: 10.1056/NEJMoa1500896. Epub 2015 Mar 17. PMID: 25776532.
23. ProCESS Investigators; Yealy DM, Kellum JA, Huang DT, Barnato AE, Weissfeld LA, Pike F, Terndrup T, Wang HE, Hou PC, LoVecchio F, Filbin MR, Shapiro NI, Angus DC. A randomized trial of protocol-based care for early septic shock. N Engl J Med. 2014 May 1;370(18):1683-93. doi: 10.1056/NEJMoa1401602. Epub 2014 Mar 18. PMID: 24635773; PMCID: PMC4101700.
24. ARISE Investigators; ANZICS Clinical Trials Group; Peake SL, Delaney A, Bailey M, Bellomo R, Cameron PA, Cooper DJ, Higgins AM, Holdgate A, Howe BD, Webb SA, Williams P. Goal-directed resuscitation for patients with early septic shock. N Engl J Med. 2014 Oct 16;371(16):1496-506. doi: 10.1056/NEJMoa1404380. Epub 2014 Oct 1. PMID: 25272316.
25. Hernández G, Teboul JL, Bakker J. Norepinephrine in septic shock. Intensive Care Med. 2019 May;45(5):687-689. doi: 10.1007/s00134-018-5499-8. Epub 2019 Jan 10. Erratum in: Intensive Care Med. 2019 Apr;45(4):561. PMID: 30631902.
26. Guinot PG, Longrois D, Kamel S, Lorne E, Dupont H. Ventriculo-Arterial Coupling Analysis Predicts the Hemodynamic Response to Norepinephrine in Hypotensive Postoperative Patients: A Prospective Observational Study. Crit Care Med. 2018 Jan;46(1):e17-e25. doi: 10.1097/CCM.0000000000002772. PMID: 29019850.
27. Vadiei N, Daley MJ, Murthy MS, Shuman CS. Impact of Norepinephrine Weight-Based Dosing Compared With Non-Weight-Based Dosing in Achieving Time to Goal Mean Arterial Pressure in Obese Patients With Septic Shock. Ann Pharmacother. 2017 Mar;51(3):194-202. doi: 10.1177/1060028016682030. Epub 2016 Nov 25. PMID: 27886982.
28. Selby AR, Khan NS, Dadashian T, Hall Nd RG. Evaluation of Dose Requirements Using Weight-Based versus Non-Weight-Based Dosing of Norepinephrine to Achieve a Goal Mean Arterial Pressure in Patients with Septic Shock. J Clin Med. 2023 Feb 8;12(4):1344. doi: 10.3390/jcm12041344. PMID: 36835880; PMCID: PMC9964536.
29. Waechter J, Kumar A, Lapinsky SE, Marshall J, Dodek P, Arabi Y, Parrillo JE, Dellinger RP, Garland A; Cooperative Antimicrobial Therapy of Septic Shock Database Research Group. Interaction between fluids and vasoactive agents on mortality in septic shock: a multicenter, observational study. Crit Care Med. 2014 Oct;42(10):2158-68. doi: 10.1097/CCM.0000000000000520. PMID: 25072761.
30. Colon Hidalgo D, Patel J, Masic D, Park D, Rech MA. Delayed vasopressor initiation is associated with increased mortality in patients with septic shock. J Crit Care. 2020 Feb;55:145-148. doi: 10.1016/j.jcrc.2019.11.004. Epub 2019 Nov 9. PMID: 31731173.
31. Udy AA, Finnis M, Jones D, Delaney A, Macdonald S, Bellomo R, Peake S; ARISE Investigators. Incidence, Patient Characteristics, Mode of Drug Delivery, and Outcomes of Septic Shock Patients Treated With Vasopressors in the Arise Trial. Shock. 2019 Oct;52(4):400-407. doi: 10.1097/SHK.0000000000001281. PMID: 30379749.
32. Permpikul C, Tongyoo S, Viarasilpa T, Trainarongsakul T, Chakorn T, Udompanturak S. Early Use of Norepinephrine in Septic Shock Resuscitation (CENSER). A Randomized Trial. Am J Respir Crit Care Med. 2019 May 1;199(9):1097-1105. doi: 10.1164/rccm.201806-1034OC. PMID: 30704260.
33. Ospina-Tascón GA, Hernandez G, Alvarez I, Calderón-Tapia LE, Manzano-Nunez R, Sánchez-Ortiz AI, Quiñones E, Ruiz-Yucuma JE, Aldana JL, Teboul JL, Cavalcanti AB, De Backer D, Bakker J. Effects of very early start of norepinephrine in patients with septic shock: a propensity score-based analysis. Crit Care. 2020 Feb 14;24(1):52. doi: 10.1186/s13054-020-2756-3. PMID: 32059682; PMCID: PMC7023737.

34. Li Y, Li H, Zhang D. Timing of norepinephrine initiation in patients with septic shock: a systematic review and meta-analysis. Crit Care. 2020 Aug 6;24(1):488. doi: 10.1186/s13054-020-03204-x. PMID: 32762765; PMCID: PMC7409707.
35. Hasegawa D, Ishisaka Y, Maeda T, Prasitlumkum N, Nishida K, Dugar S, Sato R. Prevalence and Prognosis of Sepsis-Induced Cardiomyopathy: A Systematic Review and Meta-Analysis. J Intensive Care Med. 2023 Jun 4:8850666231180526. doi: 10.1177/08850666231180526. Epub ahead of print. PMID: 37272081.
36. Annane D, Vignon P, Renault A, Bollaert PE, Charpentier C, Martin C, Troché G, Ricard JD, Nitenberg G, Papazian L, Azoulay E, Bellissant E; CATS Study Group. Norepinephrine plus dobutamine versus epinephrine alone for management of septic shock: a randomised trial. Lancet. 2007 Aug 25;370(9588):676-84. doi: 10.1016/S0140-6736(07)61344-0. Erratum in: Lancet. 2007 Sep 22;370(9592):1034. PMID: 17720019.
37. Levy B, Perez P, Perny J, Thivilier C, Gerard A. Comparison of norepinephrine-dobutamine to epinephrine for hemodynamics, lactate metabolism, and organ function variables in cardiogenic shock. A prospective, randomized pilot study. Crit Care Med. 2011 Mar;39(3):450-5. doi: 10.1097/CCM.0b013e3181ffe0eb. PMID: 21037469.
38. De Backer D, Biston P, Devriendt J, Madl C, Chochrad D, Aldecoa C, Brasseur A, Defrance P, Gottignies P, Vincent JL; SOAP II Investigators. Comparison of dopamine and norepinephrine in the treatment of shock. N Engl J Med. 2010 Mar 4;362(9):779-89. doi: 10.1056/NEJMoa0907118. PMID: 20200382.
39. Rui Q, Jiang Y, Chen M, Zhang N, Yang H, Zhou Y. Dopamine versus norepinephrine in the treatment of cardiogenic shock: A PRISMA-compliant meta-analysis. Medicine (Baltimore). 2017 Oct;96(43):e8402. doi: 10.1097/MD.0000000000008402. PMID: 29069037; PMCID: PMC5671870.
40. Bougouin W, Slimani K, Renaudier M, Binois Y, Paul M, Dumas F, Lamhaut L, Loeb T, Ortuno S, Deye N, Voicu S, Beganton F, Jost D, Mekontso-Dessap A, Marijon E, Jouven X, Aissaoui N, Cariou A; Sudden Death Expertise Center Investigators. Epinephrine versus norepinephrine in cardiac arrest patients with post-resuscitation shock. Intensive Care Med. 2022 Mar;48(3):300-310. doi: 10.1007/s00134-021-06608-7. Epub 2022 Feb 7. PMID: 35129643.
41. Cheng L, Yan J, Han S, Chen Q, Chen M, Jiang H, Lu J. Comparative efficacy of vasoactive medications in patients with septic shock: a network meta-analysis of randomized controlled trials. Crit Care. 2019 May 14;23(1):168. doi: 10.1186/s13054-019-2427-4. PMID: 31088524; PMCID: PMC6518735.
42. Law AC, Bosch NA, Peterson D, Walkey AJ. Comparison of Heart Rate After Phenylephrine vs Norepinephrine Initiation in Patients With Septic Shock and Atrial Fibrillation. Chest. 2022 Oct;162(4):796-803. doi: 10.1016/j.chest.2022.04.147. Epub 2022 May 5. PMID: 35526604; PMCID: PMC9808602.
43. Haiduc M, Radparvar S, Aitken SL, Altshuler J. Does Switching Norepinephrine to Phenylephrine in Septic Shock Complicated by Atrial Fibrillation With Rapid Ventricular Response Improve Time to Rate Control? J Intensive Care Med. 2021 Feb;36(2):191-196. doi: 10.1177/0885066619896292. Epub 2020 Jan 2. PMID: 31893966.
44. Hajjar LA, Vincent JL, Barbosa Gomes Galas FR, Rhodes A, Landoni G, Osawa EA, Melo RR, Sundin MR, Grande SM, Gaiotto FA, Pomerantzeff PM, Dallan LO, Franco RA, Nakamura RE, Lisboa LA, de Almeida JP, Gerent AM, Souza DH, Gaiane MA, Fukushima JT, Park CL, Zambolim C, Rocha Ferreira GS, Strabelli TM, Fernandes FL, Camara L, Zeferino S, Santos VG, Piccioni MA, Jatene FB, Costa Auler JO Jr, Filho RK. Vasopressin versus Norepinephrine in Patients with Vasoplegic Shock after Cardiac Surgery: The VANCS Randomized Controlled Trial. Anesthesiology. 2017 Jan;126(1):85-93. doi: 10.1097/ALN.0000000000001434. PMID: 27841822.
45. Kislitsina ON, Rich JD, Wilcox JE, Pham DT, Churyla A, Vorovich EB, Ghafourian K, Yancy CW. Shock – Classification and Pathophysiological Principles of Therapeutics. Curr Cardiol Rev. 2019;15(2):102-113. doi: 10.2174/1573403X15666181212125024. PMID: 30543176; PMCID: PMC6520577.
46. Thiele RH, Nemergut EC, Lynch C 3rd. The clinical implications of isolated alpha(1) adrenergic stimulation. Anesth Analg. 2011 Aug;113(2):297-304. doi: 10.1213/ANE.0b013e3182120ca5. Epub 2011 Apr 25. PMID: 21519053.
47. van Diepen S, Katz JN, Albert NM, Henry TD, Jacobs AK, Kapur NK, Kilic A, Menon V, Ohman EM, Sweitzer NK, Thiele H, Washam JB, Cohen MG; American Heart Association Council on Clinical Cardiology; Council on Cardiovascular and Stroke Nursing; Council on Quality of Care and Outcomes Research; and Mission: Lifeline. Contemporary Management of Cardiogenic Shock: A Scientific Statement From the American Heart Association. Circulation. 2017 Oct 17;136(16):e232-e268. doi: 10.1161/CIR.0000000000000525. Epub 2017 Sep 18. PMID: 28923988.
48. Singer M, Deutschman CS, Seymour CW, Shankar-Hari M, Annane D, Bauer M, Bellomo R, Bernard GR, Chiche JD, Coopersmith CM, Hotchkiss RS, Levy MM, Marshall JC, Martin GS, Opal SM, Rubenfeld GD, van der Poll T, Vincent JL, Angus DC. The Third International Consensus Definitions for Sepsis and Septic Shock (Sepsis-3). JAMA. 2016 Feb 23;315(8):801-10. doi: 10.1001/jama.2016.0287. PMID: 26903338; PMCID: PMC4968574.
49. Stolk RF, van der Poll T, Angus DC, van der Hoeven JG, Pickkers P, Kox M. Potentially Inadvertent Immunomodulation: Norepinephrine Use in Sepsis. Am J Respir Crit Care Med. 2016 Sep 1;194(5):550-8. doi: 10.1164/rccm.201604-0862CP. PMID: 27398737.
50. Iyer SS, Cheng G. Role of interleukin 10 transcriptional regulation in inflammation and autoimmune disease. Crit Rev Immunol. 2012;32(1):23-63. doi: 10.1615/critrevimmunol.v32.i1.30. PMID: 22428854; PMCID: PMC3410706.
51. Stolk RF, van der Pasch E, Naumann F, Schouwstra J, Bressers S, van Herwaarden AE, Gerretsen J, Schambergen R, Ruth MM, van der Hoeven JG, van Leeuwen H, Pickkers P, Kox M. Norepinephrine Dysregulates the Immune Response and Compromises Host Defense during Sepsis. Am J Respir Crit Care Med. 2020 Sep 15;202(6):830-842. doi: 10.1164/rccm.202002-0339OC. PMID: 32520577.
52. Ulf von Euler – Facts. NobelPrize.org. Nobel Prize Outreach AB 2023. Sat. 21 Oct 2023. https://www.nobelprize.org/prizes/medicine/1970/euler/facts/
53. MILLER AJ, SHIFRIN A, KAPLAN BM, GOLD H, BILLINGS A, KATZ LN. Arterenol in treatment of shock. J Am Med Assoc. 1953 Jul 25;152(13):1198-1201. doi: 10.1001/jama.1953.03690130014003. PMID: 13061238.

54. Mampuya WM, Dumont J, Lamontagne F. Norepinephrine-associated left ventricular outflow tract obstruction and systolic anterior movement. BMJ Case Rep. 2019 Dec 2;12(12):e225879. doi: 10.1136/bcr-2018-225879. PMID: 31796448; PMCID: PMC7001716.
55. Leone M, Goyer I, Levy B, Dünser MW, Asfar P, Jentzer JC. Dose of norepinephrine: the devil is in the details. Intensive Care Med. 2022 May;48(5):638-640. doi: 10.1007/s00134-022-06652-x. Epub 2022 Mar 15. PMID: 35290485.

EPINEPHRINE CITATIONS

1. Overgaard CB, Dzavík V. Inotropes and vasopressors: review of physiology and clinical use in cardiovascular disease. Circulation. 2008 Sep 2;118(10):1047-56. doi: 10.1161/CIRCULATIONAHA.107.728840. PMID: 18765387.
2. Hollenberg SM. Vasoactive drugs in circulatory shock. Am J Respir Crit Care Med. 2011 Apr 1;183(7):847-55. doi: 10.1164/rccm.201006-0972CI. Epub 2010 Nov 19. PMID: 21097695.
3. van Diepen S, Katz JN, Albert NM, Henry TD, Jacobs AK, Kapur NK, Kilic A, Menon V, Ohman EM, Sweitzer NK, Thiele H, Washam JB, Cohen MG; American Heart Association Council on Clinical Cardiology; Council on Cardiovascular and Stroke Nursing; Council on Quality of Care and Outcomes Research; and Mission: Lifeline. Contemporary Management of Cardiogenic Shock: A Scientific Statement From the American Heart Association. Circulation. 2017 Oct 17;136(16):e232-e268. doi: 10.1161/CIR.0000000000000525. Epub 2017 Sep 18. PMID: 28923988.
4. Levy B, Clere-Jehl R, Legras A, Morichau-Beauchant T, Leone M, Frederique G, Quenot JP, Kimmoun A, Cariou A, Lassus J, Harjola VP, Meziani F, Louis G, Rossignol P, Duarte K, Girerd N, Mebazaa A, Vignon P; Collaborators. Epinephrine Versus Norepinephrine for Cardiogenic Shock After Acute Myocardial Infarction. J Am Coll Cardiol. 2018 Jul 10;72(2):173-182. doi: 10.1016/j.jacc.2018.04.051. PMID: 29976291.
5. Levy B, Buzon J, Kimmoun A. Inotropes and vasopressors use in cardiogenic shock: when, which and how much? Curr Opin Crit Care. 2019 Aug;25(4):384-390. doi: 10.1097/MCC.0000000000000632. PMID: 31166204.
6. Busse LW, Barker N, Petersen C. Vasoplegic syndrome following cardiothoracic surgery-review of pathophysiology and update of treatment options. Crit Care. 2020 Feb 4;24(1):36. doi: 10.1186/s13054-020-2743-8. PMID: 32019600; PMCID: PMC7001322.
7. Bruno RR, Wolff G, Kelm M, Jung C. Pharmacological treatment of cardiogenic shock - A state of the art review. Pharmacol Ther. 2022 Dec;240:108230. doi: 10.1016/j.pharmthera.2022.108230. Epub 2022 Jun 10. PMID: 35697151.
8. Jentzer JC, Coons JC, Link CB, Schmidhofer M. Pharmacotherapy update on the use of vasopressors and inotropes in the intensive care unit. J Cardiovasc Pharmacol Ther. 2015 May;20(3):249-60. doi: 10.1177/1074248414559838. Epub 2014 Nov 28. PMID: 25432872.
9. Shabana A, Dholoo F, Banerjee P. Inotropic Agents and Vasopressors in the Treatment of Cardiogenic Shock. Curr Heart Fail Rep. 2020 Dec;17(6):438-448. doi: 10.1007/s11897-020-00493-9. Epub 2020 Oct 26. PMID: 33103204.
10. Farmakis D, Agostoni P, Baholli L, Bautin A, Comin-Colet J, Crespo-Leiro MG, Fedele F, García-Pinilla JM, Giannakoulas G, Grigioni F, Gruchała M, Gustafsson F, Harjola VP, Hasin T, Herpain A, Iliodromitis EK, Karason K, Kivikko M, Liaudet L, Ljubas-Maček J, Marini M, Masip J, Mebazaa A, Nikolaou M, Ostadal P, Pöder P, Pollesello P, Polyzogopoulou E, Pölzl G, Tschope C, Varpula M, von Lewinski D, Vrtovec B, Yilmaz MB, Zima E, Parissis J. A pragmatic approach to the use of inotropes for the management of acute and advanced heart failure: An expert panel consensus. Int J Cardiol. 2019 Dec 15;297:83-90. doi: 10.1016/j.ijcard.2019.09.005. Epub 2019 Sep 6. PMID: 31615650.
11. Sarma D, Jentzer J. Cardiogenic Shock: Pathogenesis, Classification, and Management. Critical Care Clinics. Published: July 05, 2023. doi: 10.1016/j.ccc.2023.05.001
12. Russell JA, Gordon AC, Williams MD, Boyd JH, Walley KR, Kissoon N. Vasopressor Therapy in the Intensive Care Unit. Semin Respir Crit Care Med. 2021 Feb;42(1):59-77. doi: 10.1055/s-0040-1710320. Epub 2020 Aug 20. PMID: 32802475.
13. Evans L, Rhodes A, Alhazzani W, Antonelli M, Coopersmith CM, French C, Machado FR, Mcintyre L, Ostermann M, Prescott HC, Schorr C, Simpson S, Wiersinga WJ, Alshamsi F, Angus DC, Arabi Y, Azevedo L, Beale R, Beilman G, Belley-Cote E, Burry L, Cecconi M, Centofanti J, Coz Yataco A, De Waele J, Dellinger RP, Doi K, Du B, Estenssoro E, Ferrer R, Gomersall C, Hodgson C, Møller MH, Iwashyna T, Jacob S, Kleinpell R, Klompas M, Koh Y, Kumar A, Kwizera A, Lobo S, Masur H, McGloughlin S, Mehta S, Mehta Y, Mer M, Nunnally M, Oczkowski S, Osborn T, Papathanassoglou E, Perner A, Puskarich M, Roberts J, Schweickert W, Seckel M, Sevransky J, Sprung CL, Welte T, Zimmerman J, Levy M. Surviving sepsis campaign: international guidelines for management of sepsis and septic shock 2021. Intensive Care Med. 2021 Nov;47(11):1181-1247. doi: 10.1007/s00134-021-06506-y. Epub 2021 Oct 2. PMID: 34599691; PMCID: PMC8486643.
14. Sacha GL, Bauer SR, Lat I. Vasoactive Agent Use in Septic Shock: Beyond First-Line Recommendations. Pharmacotherapy. 2019 Mar;39(3):369-381. doi: 10.1002/phar.2220. Epub 2019 Feb 7. PMID: 30644586.
15. Myburgh JA, Higgins A, Jovanovska A, Lipman J, Ramakrishnan N, Santamaria J; CAT Study investigators. A comparison of epinephrine and norepinephrine in critically ill patients. Intensive Care Med. 2008 Dec;34(12):2226-34. doi: 10.1007/s00134-008-1219-0. Epub 2008 Jul 25. PMID: 18654759.
16. Bangash MN, Kong ML, Pearse RM. Use of inotropes and vasopressor agents in critically ill patients. Br J Pharmacol. 2012 Apr;165(7):2015-33. doi: 10.1111/j.1476-5381.2011.01588.x. PMID: 21740415; PMCID: PMC3413841.
17. Levy B, Perez P, Perny J, Thivilier C, Gerard A. Comparison of norepinephrine-dobutamine to epinephrine for hemodynamics, lactate metabolism, and organ function variables in cardiogenic shock. A prospective, randomized pilot study. Crit Care Med. 2011 Mar;39(3):450-5. doi: 10.1097/CCM.0b013e3181ffe0eb. PMID: 21037469.

18. Léopold V, Gayat E, Pirracchio R, Spinar J, Parenica J, Tarvasmäki T, Lassus J, Harjola VP, Champion S, Zannad F, Valente S, Urban P, Chua HR, Bellomo R, Popovic B, Ouweneel DM, Henriques JPS, Simonis G, Lévy B, Kimmoun A, Gaudard P, Basir MB, Markota A, Adler C, Reuter H, Mebazaa A, Chouihed T. Epinephrine and short-term survival in cardiogenic shock: an individual data meta-analysis of 2583 patients. Intensive Care Med. 2018 Jun;44(6):847-856. doi: 10.1007/s00134-018-5222-9. Epub 2018 Jun 1. Erratum in: Intensive Care Med. 2018 Nov;44(11):2022-2023. PMID: 29858926.
19. Hasegawa D, Ishisaka Y, Maeda T, Prasitlumkum N, Nishida K, Dugar S, Sato R. Prevalence and Prognosis of Sepsis-Induced Cardiomyopathy: A Systematic Review and Meta-Analysis. J Intensive Care Med. 2023 Jun 4:8850666231180526. doi: 10.1177/08850666231180526. Epub ahead of print. PMID: 37272081.
20. Annane D, Vignon P, Renault A, Bollaert PE, Charpentier C, Martin C, Troché G, Ricard JD, Nitenberg G, Papazian L, Azoulay E, Bellissant E; CATS Study Group. Norepinephrine plus dobutamine versus epinephrine alone for management of septic shock: a randomised trial. Lancet. 2007 Aug 25;370(9588):676-84. doi: 10.1016/S0140-6736(07)61344-0. Erratum in: Lancet. 2007 Sep 22;370(9592):1034. PMID: 17720019.
21. Dünser MW, Festic E, Dondorp A, Kissoon N, Ganbat T, Kwizera A, Haniffa R, Baker T, Schultz MJ; Global Intensive Care Working Group of European Society of Intensive Care Medicine. Recommendations for sepsis management in resource-limited settings. Intensive Care Med. 2012 Apr;38(4):557-74. doi: 10.1007/s00134-012-2468-5. Epub 2012 Feb 14. Erratum in: Intensive Care Med. 2012 Apr;38(4):575-6. PMID: 22349419; PMCID: PMC3307996.
22. Russell JA. Vasopressor therapy in critically ill patients with shock. Intensive Care Med. 2019 Nov;45(11):1503-1517. doi: 10.1007/s00134-019-05801-z. Epub 2019 Oct 23. PMID: 31646370.
23. Kraut JA, Madias NE. Lactic acidosis. N Engl J Med. 2014 Dec 11;371(24):2309-19. doi: 10.1056/NEJMra1309483. PMID: 25494270.
24. Spiegel R, Gordon D, Marik PE. The origins of the Lacto-Bolo reflex: the mythology of lactate in sepsis. J Thorac Dis. 2020 Feb;12(Suppl 1):S48-S53. doi: 10.21037/jtd.2019.11.48. PMID: 32148925; PMCID: PMC7024759.
25. Levy B, Desebbe O, Montemont C, Gibot S. Increased aerobic glycolysis through beta2 stimulation is a common mechanism involved in lactate formation during shock states. Shock. 2008 Oct;30(4):417-21. doi: 10.1097/SHK.0b013e318167378f. PMID: 18323749.
26. Levy B, Gibot S, Franck P, Cravoisy A, Bollaert PE. Relation between muscle Na+K+ ATPase activity and raised lactate concentrations in septic shock: a prospective study. Lancet. 2005 Mar 5-11;365(9462):871-5. doi: 10.1016/S0140-6736(05)71045-X. Erratum in: Lancet. 2005 Jul 9-15;366(9480):122. PMID: 15752531.
27. Levy B, Bollaert PE, Charpentier C, Nace L, Audibert G, Bauer P, Nabet P, Larcan A. Comparison of norepinephrine and dobutamine to epinephrine for hemodynamics, lactate metabolism, and gastric tonometric variables in septic shock: a prospective, randomized study. Intensive Care Med. 1997 Mar;23(3):282-7. doi: 10.1007/s001340050329. PMID: 9083230.
28. Mahmoud KM, Ammar AS. Norepinephrine supplemented with dobutamine or epinephrine for the cardiovascular support of patients with septic shock. Indian J Crit Care Med. 2012 Apr;16(2):75-80. doi: 10.4103/0972-5229.99110. PMID: 22988361; PMCID: PMC3439782.
29. Suetrong B, Walley KR. Lactic Acidosis in Sepsis: It's Not All Anaerobic: Implications for Diagnosis and Management. Chest. 2016 Jan;149(1):252-61. doi: 10.1378/chest.15-1703. Epub 2016 Jan 6. PMID: 26378980.
30. Marik P. Lactate clearance as a target of therapy in sepsis: a flawed paradigm. OA Crit Care. 2013;1:3.
31. Hernández G, Ospina-Tascón GA, Damiani LP, Estenssoro E, Dubin A, Hurtado J, Friedman G, Castro R, Alegría L, Teboul JL, Cecconi M, Ferri G, Jibaja M, Pairumani R, Fernández P, Barahona D, Granda-Luna V, Cavalcanti AB, Bakker J; The ANDROMEDA SHOCK Investigators and the Latin America Intensive Care Network (LIVEN); Hernández G, Ospina-Tascón G, Petri Damiani L, Estenssoro E, Dubin A, Hurtado J, Friedman G, Castro R, Alegría L, Teboul JL, Cecconi M, Cecconi M, Ferri G, Jibaja M, Pairumani R, Fernández P, Barahona D, Cavalcanti AB, Bakker J, Hernández G, Alegría L, Ferri G, Rodriguez N, Holger P, Soto N, Pozo M, Bakker J, Cook D, Vincent JL, Rhodes A, Kavanagh BP, Dellinger P, Rietdijk W, Carpio D, Pavéz N, Henriquez E, Bravo S, Valenzuela ED, Vera M, Dreyse J, Oviedo V, Cid MA, Larroulet M, Petruska E, Sarabia C, Gallardo D, Sanchez JE, González H, Arancibia JM, Muñoz A, Ramirez G, Aravena F, Aquevedo A, Zambrano F, Bozinovic M, Valle F, Ramirez M, Rossel V, Muñoz F, Ceballos C, Esveile C, Carmona C, Candia E, Mendoza D, Sanchez A, Ponce D, Ponce D, Lastra J, Nahuelpán B, Fasce F, Luengo C, Medel N, Cortés C, Campassi L, Rubatto P, Horna N, Furche M, Pendino JC, Bettini L, Lovesio C, González MC, Rodruguez J, Canales H, Caminos F, Galletti C, Minoldo E, Aramburu MJ, Olmos D, Nin N, Tenzi J, Quiroga C, Lacuesta P, Gaudín A, Pais R, Silvestre A, Olivera G, Rieppi G, Berrutti D, Ochoa M, Cobos P, Vintimilla F, Ramirez V, Tobar M, García F, Picoita F, Remache N, Granda V, Paredes F, Barzallo E, Garcés P, Guerrero F, Salazar S, Torres G, Tana C, Calahorrano J, Solis F, Torres P, Herrera L, Ornes A, Peréz V, Delgado G, López A, Espinosa E, Moreira J, Salcedo B, Villacres I, Suing J, Lopez M, Gomez L, Toctaquiza G, Cadena Zapata M, Orazabal MA, Pard Espejo R, Jimenez J, Calderón A, Paredes G, Barberán JL, Moya T, Atehortua H, Sabogal R, Ortiz G, Lara A, Sanchez F, Hernán Portilla A, Dávila H, Mora JA, Calderón LE, Alvarez I, Escobar E, Bejarano A, Bustamante LA, Aldana JL. Effect of a Resuscitation Strategy Targeting Peripheral Perfusion Status vs Serum Lactate Levels on 28-Day Mortality Among Patients With Septic Shock: The ANDROMEDA-SHOCK Randomized Clinical Trial. JAMA. 2019 Feb 19;321(7):654-664. doi: 10.1001/jama.2019.0071. PMID: 30772908; PMCID: PMC6439620.
32. Prielipp RC, MacGregor DA, Royster RL, Kon ND, Hines MH, Butterworth JF 4th. Dobutamine antagonizes epinephrine's biochemical and cardiotonic effects: results of an in vitro model using human lymphocytes and a clinical study in patients recovering from cardiac surgery. Anesthesiology. 1998 Jul;89(1):49-57. doi: 10.1097/00000542-199807000-00010. PMID: 9667293.
33. Bassi E, Park M, Azevedo LC. Therapeutic strategies for high-dose vasopressor-dependent shock. Crit Care Res Pract. 2013;2013:654708. doi: 10.1155/2013/654708. Epub 2013 Sep 15. PMID: 24151551; PMCID: PMC3787628
34. Epinephrine injection [package insert]. Bridgewater, NJ; Amneal; January 2021.

35. Britannica, The Editors of Encyclopaedia. "John Jacob Abel". Encyclopedia Britannica, 22 May. 2023, https://www.britannica.com/biography/John-Jacob-Abel. Accessed 8 September 2023.
36. Hollenberg SM. Vasopressor support in septic shock. Chest. 2007 Nov;132(5):1678-87. doi: 10.1378/chest.07-0291. PMID: 17998371.

PHENYLEPHRINE CITATIONS

1. Morelli A, Ertmer C, Rehberg S, Lange M, Orecchioni A, Laderchi A, Bachetoni A, D'Alessandro M, Van Aken H, Pietropaoli P, Westphal M. Phenylephrine versus norepinephrine for initial hemodynamic support of patients with septic shock: a randomized, controlled trial. Crit Care. 2008;12(6):R143. doi: 10.1186/cc7121. Epub 2008 Nov 18. PMID: 19017409; PMCID: PMC2646303.
2. Morelli A, Lange M, Ertmer C, Dünser M, Rehberg S, Bachetoni A, D'Alessandro M, Van Aken H, Guarracino F, Pietropaoli P, Traber DL, Westphal M. Short-term effects of phenylephrine on systemic and regional hemodynamics in patients with septic shock: a crossover pilot study. Shock. 2008 Apr;29(4):446-51. doi: 10.1097/shk.0b013e31815810ff. PMID: 17885646.
3. Thiele RH, Nemergut EC, Lynch C 3rd. The clinical implications of isolated alpha(1) adrenergic stimulation. Anesth Analg. 2011 Aug;113(2):297-304. doi: 10.1213/ANE.0b013e3182120ca5. Epub 2011 Apr 25. PMID: 21519053.
4. Jensen BC, Swigart PM, Laden ME, DeMarco T, Hoopes C, Simpson PC. The alpha-1D Is the predominant alpha-1-adrenergic receptor subtype in human epicardial coronary arteries. J Am Coll Cardiol. 2009 Sep 22;54(13):1137-45. doi: 10.1016/j.jacc.2009.05.056. PMID: 19761933; PMCID: PMC2812029.
5. Kislitsina ON, Rich JD, Wilcox JE, Pham DT, Churyla A, Vorovich EB, Ghafourian K, Yancy CW. Shock – Classification and Pathophysiological Principles of Therapeutics. Curr Cardiol Rev. 2019;15(2):102-113. doi: 10.2174/1573403X15666181212125024. PMID: 30543176; PMCID: PMC6520577.
6. Russell JA. Vasopressor therapy in critically ill patients with shock. Intensive Care Med. 2019 Nov;45(11):1503-1517. doi: 10.1007/s00134-019-05801-z. Epub 2019 Oct 23. PMID: 31646370.
7. Dellinger RP, Levy MM, Carlet JM, Bion J, Parker MM, Jaeschke R, Reinhart K, Angus DC, Brun-Buisson C, Beale R, Calandra T, Dhainaut JF, Gerlach H, Harvey M, Marini JJ, Marshall J, Ranieri M, Ramsay G, Sevransky J, Thompson BT, Townsend S, Vender JS, Zimmerman JL, Vincent JL; International Surviving Sepsis Campaign Guidelines Committee; American Association of Critical-Care Nurses; American College of Chest Physicians; American College of Emergency Physicians; Canadian Critical Care Society; European Society of Clinical Microbiology and Infectious Diseases; European Society of Intensive Care Medicine; European Respiratory Society; International Sepsis Forum; Japanese Association for Acute Medicine; Japanese Society of Intensive Care Medicine; Society of Critical Care Medicine; Society of Hospital Medicine; Surgical Infection Society; World Federation of Societies of Intensive and Critical Care Medicine. Surviving Sepsis Campaign: international guidelines for management of severe sepsis and septic shock: 2008. Crit Care Med. 2008 Jan;36(1):296-327. doi: 10.1097/01.CCM.0000298158.12101.41. Erratum in: Crit Care Med. 2008 Apr;36(4):1394-6. PMID: 18158437.
8. Vail E, Gershengorn HB, Hua M, Walkey AJ, Rubenfeld G, Wunsch H. Association Between US Norepinephrine Shortage and Mortality Among Patients With Septic Shock. JAMA. 2017 Apr 11;317(14):1433-1442. doi: 10.1001/jama.2017.2841. PMID: 28322415.
9. Arishi H, AlQahtani S, Tamim H, Sadat M, Alenezi FZ, Bin Humaid F, AlWehaibi W, Arabi YM. Combination of norepinephrine with phenylephrine versus norepinephrine with vasopressin in critically ill patients with septic shock: A retrospective study. J Crit Care. 2022 Dec;72:154121. doi: 10.1016/j.jcrc.2022.154121. Epub 2022 Jul 28. PMID: 35908329.
10. Haiduc M, Radparvar S, Aitken SL, Altshuler J. Does Switching Norepinephrine to Phenylephrine in Septic Shock Complicated by Atrial Fibrillation With Rapid Ventricular Response Improve Time to Rate Control? J Intensive Care Med. 2021 Feb;36(2):191-196. doi: 10.1177/0885066619896292. Epub 2020 Jan 2. PMID: 31893966.
11. Law AC, Bosch NA, Peterson D, Walkey AJ. Comparison of Heart Rate After Phenylephrine vs Norepinephrine Initiation in Patients With Septic Shock and Atrial Fibrillation. Chest. 2022 Oct;162(4):796-803. doi: 10.1016/j.chest.2022.04.147. Epub 2022 May 5. PMID: 35526604; PMCID: PMC9808602.
12. Evans L, Rhodes A, Alhazzani W, Antonelli M, Coopersmith CM, French C, Machado FR, Mcintyre L, Ostermann M, Prescott HC, Schorr C, Simpson S, Wiersinga WJ, Alshamsi F, Angus DC, Arabi Y, Azevedo L, Beale R, Beilman G, Belley-Cote E, Burry L, Cecconi M, Centofanti J, Coz Yataco A, De Waele J, Dellinger RP, Doi K, Du B, Estenssoro E, Ferrer R, Gomersall C, Hodgson C, Møller MH, Iwashyna T, Jacob S, Kleinpell R, Klompas M, Koh Y, Kumar A, Kwizera A, Lobo S, Masur H, McGloughlin S, Mehta S, Mehta Y, Mer M, Nunnally M, Oczkowski S, Osborn T, Papathanassoglou E, Perner A, Puskarich M, Roberts J, Schweickert W, Seckel M, Sevransky J, Sprung CL, Welte T, Zimmerman J, Levy M. Surviving sepsis campaign: international guidelines for management of sepsis and septic shock 2021. Intensive Care Med. 2021 Nov;47(11):1181-1247. doi: 10.1007/s00134-021-06506-y. Epub 2021 Oct 2. PMID: 34599691; PMCID: PMC8486643.
13. Dellinger RP, Levy MM, Rhodes A, Annane D, Gerlach H, Opal SM, Sevransky JE, Sprung CL, Douglas IS, Jaeschke R, Osborn TM, Nunnally ME, Townsend SR, Reinhart K, Kleinpell RM, Angus DC, Deutschman CS, Machado FR, Rubenfeld GD, Webb SA, Beale RJ, Vincent JL, Moreno R; Surviving Sepsis Campaign Guidelines Committee including the Pediatric Subgroup. Surviving sepsis campaign: international guidelines for management of severe sepsis and septic shock: 2012. Crit Care Med. 2013 Feb;41(2):580-637. doi: 10.1097/CCM.0b013e31827e83af. PMID: 23353941.
14. Rhodes A, Evans LE, Alhazzani W, Levy MM, Antonelli M, Ferrer R, Kumar A, Sevransky JE, Sprung CL, Nunnally ME, Rochwerg B, Rubenfeld GD, Angus DC, Annane D, Beale RJ, Bellinghan GJ, Bernard GR, Chiche JD, Coopersmith C, De Backer DP, French CJ, Fujishima S, Gerlach H, Hidalgo JL, Hollenberg SM, Jones AE, Karnad DR, Kleinpell RM, Koh Y, Lisboa TC, Machado FR, Marini JJ, Marshall JC, Mazuski JE, McIntyre LA, McLean AS,

Mehta S, Moreno RP, Myburgh J, Navalesi P, Nishida O, Osborn TM, Perner A, Plunkett CM, Ranieri M, Schorr CA, Seckel MA, Seymour CW, Shieh L, Shukri KA, Simpson SQ, Singer M, Thompson BT, Townsend SR, Van der Poll T, Vincent JL, Wiersinga WJ, Zimmerman JL, Dellinger RP. Surviving Sepsis Campaign: International Guidelines for Management of Sepsis and Septic Shock: 2016. Intensive Care Med. 2017 Mar;43(3):304-377. doi: 10.1007/s00134-017-4683-6. Epub 2017 Jan 18. PMID: 28101605.

15. Haley JH, Sinak LJ, Tajik AJ, Ommen SR, Oh JK. Dynamic left ventricular outflow tract obstruction in acute coronary syndromes: an important cause of new systolic murmur and cardiogenic shock. Mayo Clin Proc. 1999 Sep;74(9):901-6. doi: 10.4065/74.9.901. PMID: 10488794.

16. BRAUNWALD E, EBERT PA. Hemodynamic alterations in idiopathic hypertrophic subaortic stenosis induced by sympathomimetic drugs. Am J Cardiol. 1962 Oct;10:489-95. doi: 10.1016/0002-9149(62)90373-9. PMID: 14015086.

17. American College of Cardiology Foundation/American Heart Association Task Force on Practice Guidelines; American Association for Thoracic Surgery; American Society of Echocardiography; American Society of Nuclear Cardiology; Heart Failure Society of America; Heart Rhythm Society; Society for Cardiovascular Angiography and Interventions; Society of Thoracic Surgeons; Gersh BJ, Maron BJ, Bonow RO, Dearani JA, Fifer MA, Link MS, Naidu SS, Nishimura RA, Ommen SR, Rakowski H, Seidman CE, Towbin JA, Udelson JE, Yancy CW. 2011 ACCF/AHA guideline for the diagnosis and treatment of hypertrophic cardiomyopathy: executive summary: a report of the American College of Cardiology Foundation/American Heart Association Task Force on Practice Guidelines. J Thorac Cardiovasc Surg. 2011 Dec;142(6):1303-38. doi: 10.1016/j.jtcvs.2011.10.019. PMID: 22093712.

18. Authors/Task Force members; Elliott PM, Anastasakis A, Borger MA, Borggrefe M, Cecchi F, Charron P, Hagege AA, Lafont A, Limongelli G, Mahrholdt H, McKenna WJ, Mogensen J, Nihoyannopoulos P, Nistri S, Pieper PG, Pieske B, Rapezzi C, Rutten FH, Tillmanns C, Watkins H. 2014 ESC Guidelines on diagnosis and management of hypertrophic cardiomyopathy: the Task Force for the Diagnosis and Management of Hypertrophic Cardiomyopathy of the European Society of Cardiology (ESC). Eur Heart J. 2014 Oct 14;35(39):2733-79. doi: 10.1093/eurheartj/ehu284. Epub 2014 Aug 29. PMID: 25173338.

19. Goertz AW, Lindner KH, Seefelder C, Schirmer U, Beyer M, Georgieff M. Effect of phenylephrine bolus administration on global left ventricular function in patients with coronary artery disease and patients with valvular aortic stenosis. Anesthesiology. 1993 May;78(5):834-41. doi: 10.1097/00000542-199305000-00005. PMID: 8489054.

20. van Diepen S, Katz JN, Albert NM, Henry TD, Jacobs AK, Kapur NK, Kilic A, Menon V, Ohman EM, Sweitzer NK, Thiele H, Washam JB, Cohen MG; American Heart Association Council on Clinical Cardiology; Council on Cardiovascular and Stroke Nursing; Council on Quality of Care and Outcomes Research; and Mission: Lifeline. Contemporary Management of Cardiogenic Shock: A Scientific Statement From the American Heart Association. Circulation. 2017 Oct 17;136(16):e232-e268. doi: 10.1161/CIR.0000000000000525. Epub 2017 Sep 18. PMID: 28923988.

21. McPherson KL, Kovacic Scherrer NL, Hays WB, Greco AR, Garavaglia JM. A Review of Push-Dose Vasopressors in the Peri-operative and Critical Care Setting. J Pharm Pract. 2023 Aug;36(4):925-932. doi: 10.1177/08971900221096967. Epub 2022 Apr 22. PMID: 35459405.

22. Kubena A, Weston S, Alvey H. Push-dose vasopressors in the Emergency Department: a narrative review. J Emerg Crit Care Med 2022;6:22. doi: 10.21037/jeccm-21-98

23. Hawn JM, Bauer SR, Yerke J, Li M, Wang X, Reddy AJ, Mireles-Cabodevila E, Sacha GL. Effect of Phenylephrine Push Before Continuous Infusion Norepinephrine in Patients With Septic Shock. Chest. 2021 May;159(5):1875-1883. doi: 10.1016/j.chest.2020.11.051. Epub 2020 Dec 13. PMID: 33316239.

24. Hajjar LA, Vincent JL, Barbosa Gomes Galas FR, Rhodes A, Landoni G, Osawa EA, Melo RR, Sundin MR, Grande SM, Gaiotto FA, Pomerantzeff PM, Dallan LO, Franco RA, Nakamura RE, Lisboa LA, de Almeida JP, Gerent AM, Souza DH, Gaiane MA, Fukushima JT, Park CL, Zambolim C, Rocha Ferreira GS, Strabelli TM, Fernandes FL, Camara L, Zeferino S, Santos VG, Piccioni MA, Jatene FB, Costa Auler JO Jr, Filho RK. Vasopressin versus Norepinephrine in Patients with Vasoplegic Shock after Cardiac Surgery: The VANCS Randomized Controlled Trial. Anesthesiology. 2017 Jan;126(1):85-93. doi: 10.1097/ALN.0000000000001434. PMID: 27841822.

25. Levy B, Fritz C, Tahon E, Jacquot A, Auchet T, Kimmoun A. Vasoplegia treatments: the past, the present, and the future. Crit Care. 2018 Feb 27;22(1):52. doi: 10.1186/s13054-018-1967-3. PMID: 29486781; PMCID: PMC6389278.

26. Levine AR, Meyer MJ, Bittner EA, Berg S, Kalman R, Stanislaus AB, Ryan C, Ball SA, Eikermann M. Oral midodrine treatment accelerates the liberation of intensive care unit patients from intravenous vasopressor infusions. J Crit Care. 2013 Oct;28(5):756-62. doi: 10.1016/j.jcrc.2013.05.021. Epub 2013 Jul 8. PMID: 23845791.

27. Keys A, Violante A. THE CARDIO-CIRCULATORY EFFECTS IN MAN OF NEO-SYNEPHRIN (1-alpha-hydroxy-beta-methylamino-3-hydroxy-ethylbenzene hydrochloride). J Clin Invest. 1942 Jan;21(1):1-12. doi: 10.1172/JCI101270. PMID: 16694882; PMCID: PMC435110.

28. PHENYLEPHRINE HYDROCHLORIDE package insert, Eatontown, NJ: West-ward, Inc.; 2012.

VASOPRESSIN

1. Vail EA, Gershengorn HB, Hua M, Walkey AJ, Wunsch H. Epidemiology of Vasopressin Use for Adults with Septic Shock. Ann Am Thorac Soc. 2016 Oct;13(10):1760-1767. doi: 10.1513/AnnalsATS.201604-259OC. PMID: 27404213; PMCID: PMC5122493.

2. "Vasopressin Injection, USP." FDA.gov, U.S. Food and Drug Administration, 2023.

3. Holmes CL, Patel BM, Russell JA, Walley KR. Physiology of vasopressin relevant to management of septic shock. Chest. 2001 Sep;120(3):989-1002. doi: 10.1378/chest.120.3.989. PMID: 11555538.

4. Landry DW, Levin HR, Gallant EM, Ashton RC Jr, Seo S, D'Alessandro D, Oz MC, Oliver JA. Vasopressin deficiency contributes to the vasodilation of septic shock. Circulation. 1997 Mar 4;95(5):1122-5. doi: 10.1161/01.cir.95.5.1122. PMID: 9054839.
5. Sharshar T, Carlier R, Blanchard A, Feydy A, Gray F, Paillard M, Raphael JC, Gajdos P, Annane D. Depletion of neurohypophyseal content of vasopressin in septic shock. Crit Care Med. 2002 Mar;30(3):497-500. doi: 10.1097/00003246-200203000-00001. PMID: 11990905.
6. Russell JA, Walley KR, Singer J, Gordon AC, Hébert PC, Cooper DJ, Holmes CL, Mehta S, Granton JT, Storms MM, Cook DJ, Presneill JJ, Ayers D; VASST Investigators. Vasopressin versus norepinephrine infusion in patients with septic shock. N Engl J Med. 2008 Feb 28;358(9):877-87. doi: 10.1056/NEJMoa067373. PMID: 18305265.
7. Argenziano M, Chen JM, Choudhri AF, Cullinane S, Garfein E, Weinberg AD, Smith CR Jr, Rose EA, Landry DW, Oz MC. Management of vasodilatory shock after cardiac surgery: identification of predisposing factors and use of a novel pressor agent. J Thorac Cardiovasc Surg. 1998 Dec;116(6):973-80. doi: 10.1016/S0022-5223(98)70049-2. PMID: 9832689.
8. Hajjar LA, Vincent JL, Barbosa Gomes Galas FR, Rhodes A, Landoni G, Osawa EA, Melo RR, Sundin MR, Grande SM, Gaiotto FA, Pomerantzeff PM, Dallan LO, Franco RA, Nakamura RE, Lisboa LA, de Almeida JP, Gerent AM, Souza DH, Gaiane MA, Fukushima JT, Park CL, Zambolim C, Rocha Ferreira GS, Strabelli TM, Fernandes FL, Camara L, Zeferino S, Santos VG, Piccioni MA, Jatene FB, Costa Auler JO Jr, Filho RK. Vasopressin versus Norepinephrine in Patients with Vasoplegic Shock after Cardiac Surgery: The VANCS Randomized Controlled Trial. Anesthesiology. 2017 Jan;126(1):85-93. doi: 10.1097/ALN.0000000000001434. PMID: 27841822.
9. Möhring J, Glänzer K, Maciel JA Jr, Düsing R, Kramer HJ, Arbogast R, Koch-Weser J. Greatly enhanced pressor response to antidiuretic hormone in patients with impaired cardiovascular reflexes due to idiopathic orthostatic hypotension. J Cardiovasc Pharmacol. 1980 Jul-Aug;2(4):367-76. doi: 10.1097/00005344-198007000-00004. PMID: 6156335.
10. Graybiel A, Glendy RE. Circulatory effects following the intravenous administration of pitressin in normal persons and in patients with hypertension and angina pectoris. Am Heart J 1941;21(4):481–9. doi:10.1016/S0002-8703(41)90649-X.
11. Malay MB, Ashton RC Jr, Landry DW, Townsend RN. Low-dose vasopressin in the treatment of vasodilatory septic shock. J Trauma. 1999 Oct;47(4):699-703; discussion 703-5. doi: 10.1097/00005373-199910000-00014. PMID: 10528604.
12. Patel BM, Chittock DR, Russell JA, Walley KR. Beneficial effects of short-term vasopressin infusion during severe septic shock. Anesthesiology. 2002 Mar;96(3):576-82. doi: 10.1097/00000542-200203000-00011. PMID: 11873030.
13. Dünser MW, Mayr AJ, Ulmer H, Knotzer H, Sumann G, Pajk W, Friesenecker B, Hasibeder WR. Arginine vasopressin in advanced vasodilatory shock: a prospective, randomized, controlled study. Circulation. 2003 May 13;107(18):2313-9. doi: 10.1161/01.CIR.0000066692.71008.BB. Epub 2003 May 5. PMID: 12732600.
14. Annane D, Renault A, Brun-Buisson C, Megarbane B, Quenot JP, Siami S, Cariou A, Forceville X, Schwebel C, Martin C, Timsit JF, Misset B, Ali Benali M, Colin G, Souweine B, Asehnoune K, Mercier E, Chimot L, Charpentier C, François B, Boulain T, Petitpas F, Constantin JM, Dhonneur G, Baudin F, Combes A, Bohé J, Loriferne JF, Amathieu R, Cook F, Slama M, Leroy O, Capellier G, Dargent A, Hissem T, Maxime V, Bellissant E; CRICS-TRIGGERSEP Network. Hydrocortisone plus Fludrocortisone for Adults with Septic Shock. N Engl J Med. 2018 Mar 1;378(9):809-818. doi: 10.1056/NEJMoa1705716. PMID: 29490185.
15. Venkatesh B, Finfer S, Cohen J, Rajbhandari D, Arabi Y, Bellomo R, Billot L, Correa M, Glass P, Harward M, Joyce C, Li Q, McArthur C, Perner A, Rhodes A, Thompson K, Webb S, Myburgh J; ADRENAL Trial Investigators and the Australian–New Zealand Intensive Care Society Clinical Trials Group. Adjunctive Glucocorticoid Therapy in Patients with Septic Shock. N Engl J Med. 2018 Mar 1;378(9):797-808. doi: 10.1056/NEJMoa1705835. Epub 2018 Jan 19. PMID: 29347874.
16. Russell JA, Walley KR, Gordon AC, Cooper DJ, Hébert PC, Singer J, Holmes CL, Mehta S, Granton JT, Storms MM, Cook DJ, Presneill JJ; Dieter Ayers for the Vasopressin and Septic Shock Trial Investigators. Interaction of vasopressin infusion, corticosteroid treatment, and mortality of septic shock. Crit Care Med. 2009 Mar;37(3):811-8. doi: 10.1097/CCM.0b013e3181961ace. PMID: 19237882.
17. Gordon AC, Mason AJ, Thirunavukkarasu N, Perkins GD, Cecconi M, Cepkova M, Pogson DG, Aya HD, Anjum A, Frazier GJ, Santhakumaran S, Ashby D, Brett SJ; VANISH Investigators. Effect of Early Vasopressin vs Norepinephrine on Kidney Failure in Patients With Septic Shock: The VANISH Randomized Clinical Trial. JAMA. 2016 Aug 2;316(5):509-18. doi: 10.1001/jama.2016.10485. PMID: 27483065.
18. Evans L, Rhodes A, Alhazzani W, Antonelli M, Coopersmith CM, French C, Machado FR, Mcintyre L, Ostermann M, Prescott HC, Schorr C, Simpson S, Wiersinga WJ, Alshamsi F, Angus DC, Arabi Y, Azevedo L, Beale R, Beilman G, Belley-Cote E, Burry L, Cecconi M, Centofanti J, Coz Yataco A, De Waele J, Dellinger RP, Doi K, Du B, Estenssoro E, Ferrer R, Gomersall C, Hodgson C, Møller MH, Iwashyna T, Jacob S, Kleinpell R, Klompas M, Koh Y, Kumar A, Kwizera A, Lobo S, Masur H, McGloughlin S, Mehta S, Mehta Y, Mer M, Nunnally M, Oczkowski S, Osborn T, Papathanassoglou E, Perner A, Puskarich M, Roberts J, Schweickert W, Seckel M, Sevransky J, Sprung CL, Welte T, Zimmerman J, Levy M. Surviving sepsis campaign: international guidelines for management of sepsis and septic shock 2021. Intensive Care Med. 2021 Nov;47(11):1181-1247. doi: 10.1007/s00134-021-06506-y. Epub 2021 Oct 2. PMID: 34599691; PMCID: PMC8486643.
19. Hajjar LA, Zambolim C, Belletti A, de Almeida JP, Gordon AC, Oliveira G, Park CHL, Fukushima JT, Rizk SI, Szeles TF, Dos Santos Neto NC, Filho RK, Galas FRBG, Landoni G. Vasopressin Versus Norepinephrine for the Management of Septic Shock in Cancer Patients: The VANCS II Randomized Clinical Trial. Crit Care Med. 2019 Dec;47(12):1743-1750. doi: 10.1097/CCM.0000000000004023. PMID: 31609774.

20. Morales DL, Garrido MJ, Madigan JD, Helman DN, Faber J, Williams MR, Landry DW, Oz MC. A double-blind randomized trial: prophylactic vasopressin reduces hypotension after cardiopulmonary bypass. Ann Thorac Surg. 2003 Mar;75(3):926-30. doi: 10.1016/s0003-4975(02)04408-9. PMID: 12645718.
21. Garcia B, Legrand M. Adjunctive vasopressors in distributive shock: How soon is early? Crit Care. 2023 May 30;27(1):210. doi: 10.1186/s13054-023-04500-y. PMID: 37254175; PMCID: PMC10230760.
22. Stolk RF, van der Poll T, Angus DC, van der Hoeven JG, Pickkers P, Kox M. Potentially Inadvertent Immunomodulation: Norepinephrine Use in Sepsis. Am J Respir Crit Care Med. 2016 Sep 1;194(5):550-8. doi: 10.1164/rccm.201604-0862CP. PMID: 27398737.
23. Sacha GL, Lam SW, Wang L, Duggal A, Reddy AJ, Bauer SR. Association of Catecholamine Dose, Lactate, and Shock Duration at Vasopressin Initiation With Mortality in Patients With Septic Shock. Crit Care Med. 2022 Apr 1;50(4):614-623. doi: 10.1097/CCM.0000000000005317. PMID: 34582425.
24. Young PJ, Delaney A, Venkatesh B. Vasopressin in septic shock: what we know and where to next? Intensive Care Med. 2019 Jun;45(6):902-903. doi: 10.1007/s00134-019-05642-w. Epub 2019 May 13. PMID: 31087112.
25. Wallace AW, Tunin CM, Shoukas AA. Effects of vasopressin on pulmonary and systemic vascular mechanics. Am J Physiol. 1989 Oct;257(4 Pt 2):H1228-34. doi: 10.1152/ajpheart.1989.257.4.H1228. PMID: 2801982.
26. Evora PR, Pearson PJ, Schaff HV. Arginine vasopressin induces endothelium-dependent vasodilatation of the pulmonary artery. V1-receptor-mediated production of nitric oxide. Chest. 1993 Apr;103(4):1241-5. doi: 10.1378/chest.103.4.1241. PMID: 8131474.
27. Luckner G, Mayr VD, Jochberger S, Wenzel V, Ulmer H, Hasibeder WR, Dünser MW. Comparison of two dose regimens of arginine vasopressin in advanced vasodilatory shock. Crit Care Med. 2007 Oct;35(10):2280-5. doi: 10.1097/01.ccm.0000281853.50661.23. PMID: 17944015.
28. Currigan DA, Hughes RJ, Wright CE, Angus JA, Soeding PF. Vasoconstrictor responses to vasopressor agents in human pulmonary and radial arteries: an in vitro study. Anesthesiology. 2014 Nov;121(5):930-6. doi: 10.1097/ALN.0000000000000430. PMID: 25198173.
29. Tayama E, Ueda T, Shojima T, Akasu K, Oda T, Fukunaga S, Akashi H, Aoyagi S. Arginine vasopressin is an ideal drug after cardiac surgery for the management of low systemic vascular resistant hypotension concomitant with pulmonary hypertension. Interact Cardiovasc Thorac Surg. 2007 Dec;6(6):715-9. doi: 10.1510/icvts.2007.159624. Epub 2007 Aug 17. PMID: 17704123.
30. Jeon Y, Ryu JH, Lim YJ, Kim CS, Bahk JH, Yoon SZ, Choi JY. Comparative hemodynamic effects of vasopressin and norepinephrine after milrinone-induced hypotension in off-pump coronary artery bypass surgical patients. Eur J Cardiothorac Surg. 2006 Jun;29(6):952-6. doi: 10.1016/j.ejcts.2006.02.032. Epub 2006 May 3. PMID: 16675238.
31. Yimin H, Xiaoyu L, Yuping H, Weiyan L, Ning L. The effect of vasopressin on the hemodynamics in CABG patients. J Cardiothorac Surg. 2013 Mar 16;8:49. doi: 10.1186/1749-8090-8-49. PMID: 23497457; PMCID: PMC3610232.
32. Boyd JH, Holmes CL, Wang Y, Roberts H, Walley KR. Vasopressin decreases sepsis-induced pulmonary inflammation through the V2R. Resuscitation. 2008 Nov;79(2):325-31. doi: 10.1016/j.resuscitation.2008.07.006. PMID: 18951104.
33. Gordon AC, Russell JA, Walley KR, Singer J, Ayers D, Storms MM, Holmes CL, Hébert PC, Cooper DJ, Mehta S, Granton JT, Cook DJ, Presneill JJ. The effects of vasopressin on acute kidney injury in septic shock. Intensive Care Med. 2010 Jan;36(1):83-91. doi: 10.1007/s00134-009-1687-x. Epub 2009 Oct 20. PMID: 19841897.
34. Nagendran M, Russell JA, Walley KR, Brett SJ, Perkins GD, Hajjar L, Mason AJ, Ashby D, Gordon AC. Vasopressin in septic shock: an individual patient data meta-analysis of randomised controlled trials. Intensive Care Med. 2019 Jun;45(6):844-855. doi: 10.1007/s00134-019-05620-2. Epub 2019 May 6. PMID: 31062052.
35. Rydz AC, Elefritz JL, Conroy M, Disney KA, Miller CJ, Porter K, Doepker BA. EARLY INITIATION OF VASOPRESSIN REDUCES ORGAN FAILURE AND MORTALITY IN SEPTIC SHOCK. Shock. 2022 Oct 1;58(4):269-274. doi: 10.1097/SHK.0000000000001978. Epub 2022 Aug 16. PMID: 36018257.
36. Fox AW, May RE, Mitch WE. Comparison of peptide and nonpeptide receptor-mediated responses in rat tail artery. J Cardiovasc Pharmacol. 1992 Aug;20(2):282-9. doi: 10.1097/00005344-199208000-00014. PMID: 1381020.
37. Dunser MW, Wenzel V, Mayr AJ, Hasibeder WR. Management of vasodilatory shock: defining the role of arginine vasopressin. Drugs. 2003;63(3):237-56. doi: 10.2165/00003495-200363030-00001. PMID: 12534330.
38. Mutlu GM, Factor P. Role of vasopressin in the management of septic shock. Intensive Care Med. 2004 Jul;30(7):1276-91. doi: 10.1007/s00134-004-2283-8. Epub 2004 Apr 21. PMID: 15103461.
39. Turner DW, Attridge RL, Hughes DW. Vasopressin Associated With an Increase in Return of Spontaneous Circulation in Acidotic Cardiopulmonary Arrest Patients. Ann Pharmacother. 2014 Aug;48(8):986-991. doi: 10.1177/1060028014537037. Epub 2014 May 28. PMID: 24871568.
40. Bauer SR, Sacha GL, Siuba MT, Lam SW, Reddy AJ, Duggal A, Vachharajani V. Association of Arterial pH With Hemodynamic Response to Vasopressin in Patients With Septic Shock: An Observational Cohort Study. Crit Care Explor. 2022 Feb 8;4(2):e0634. doi: 10.1097/CCE.0000000000000634. PMID: 35156051; PMCID: PMC8826954.
41. Jaber S, Paugam C, Futier E, Lefrant JY, Lasocki S, Lescot T, Pottecher J, Demoule A, Ferrandière M, Asehnoune K, Dellamonica J, Velly L, Abback PS, de Jong A, Brunot V, Belafia F, Roquilly A, Chanques G, Muller L, Constantin JM, Bertet H, Klouche K, Molinari N, Jung B; BICAR-ICU Study Group. Sodium bicarbonate therapy for patients with severe metabolic acidaemia in the intensive care unit (BICAR-ICU): a multicentre, open-label, randomised controlled, phase 3 trial. Lancet. 2018 Jul 7;392(10141):31-40. doi: 10.1016/S0140-6736(18)31080-8. Epub 2018 Jun 14. Erratum in: Lancet. 2018 Dec 8;392(10163):2440. PMID: 29910040.
42. Garcia-Tsao G, Abraldes JG, Berzigotti A, Bosch J. Portal hypertensive bleeding in cirrhosis: Risk stratification, diagnosis, and management: 2016 practice guidance by the American Association for the study of liver diseases. Hepatology. 2017 Jan;65(1):310-335. doi: 10.1002/hep.28906. Epub 2016 Dec 1. Erratum in: Hepatology. 2017 Jul;66(1):304. PMID: 27786365.

43. Terés J, Planas R, Panes J, Salmeron JM, Mas A, Bosch J, Llorente C, Viver J, Feu F, Rodés J. Vasopressin/ nitroglycerin infusion vs. esophageal tamponade in the treatment of acute variceal bleeding: a randomized controlled trial. Hepatology. 1990 Jun;11(6):964-8. doi: 10.1002/hep.1840110609. PMID: 2114350.

44. Jiang L, Sheng Y, Feng X, Wu J. The effects and safety of vasopressin receptor agonists in patients with septic shock: a meta-analysis and trial sequential analysis. Crit Care. 2019 Mar 14;23(1):91. doi: 10.1186/ s13054-019-2362-4. PMID: 30871607; PMCID: PMC6419432.

45. Ferenchick H, Cemalovic N, Ferguson N, Dicpinigaitis PV. Diabetes Insipidus After Discontinuation of Vasopressin Infusion for Treatment of Shock. Crit Care Med. 2019 Dec;47(12):e1008-e1013. doi: 10.1097/ CCM.0000000000004045. PMID: 31567344; PMCID: PMC7086483.

46. Link MS, Berkow LC, Kudenchuk PJ, Halperin HR, Hess EP, Moitra VK, Neumar RW, O'Neil BJ, Paxton JH, Silvers SM, White RD, Yannopoulos D, Donnino MW. Part 7: Adult Advanced Cardiovascular Life Support: 2015 American Heart Association Guidelines Update for Cardiopulmonary Resuscitation and Emergency Cardiovascular Care. Circulation. 2015 Nov 3;132(18 Suppl 2):S444-64. doi: 10.1161/CIR.0000000000000261. Erratum in: Circulation. 2015 Dec 15;132(24):e385. PMID: 26472995.

47. Yan W, Dong W, Song X, Zhou W, Chen Z. Therapeutic effects of vasopressin on cardiac arrest: a systematic review and meta-analysis. BMJ Open. 2023 Apr 17;13(4):e065061. doi: 10.1136/bmjopen-2022-065061. PMID: 37068900; PMCID: PMC10111914.

48. Mukoyama T, Kinoshita K, Nagao K, Tanjoh K. Reduced effectiveness of vasopressin in repeated doses for patients undergoing prolonged cardiopulmonary resuscitation. Resuscitation. 2009 Jul;80(7):755-61. doi: 10.1016/ j.resuscitation.2009.04.005. Epub 2009 May 14. PMID: 19446387.

49. Andersen LW, Isbye D, Kjærgaard J, Kristensen CM, Darling S, Zwisler ST, Fisker S, Schmidt JC, Kirkegaard H, Grejs AM, Rossau JRG, Larsen JM, Rasmussen BS, Riddersholm S, Iversen K, Schultz M, Nielsen JL, Løfgren B, Lauridsen KG, Sølling C, Pælestik K, Kjærgaard AG, Due-Rasmussen D, Folke F, Charlot MG, Jepsen RMHG, Wiberg S, Donnino M, Kurth T, Høybye M, Sindberg B, Holmberg MJ, Granfeldt A. Effect of Vasopressin and Methylprednisolone vs Placebo on Return of Spontaneous Circulation in Patients With In-Hospital Cardiac Arrest: A Randomized Clinical Trial. JAMA. 2021 Oct 26;326(16):1586-1594. doi: 10.1001/jama.2021.16628. PMID: 34587236; PMCID: PMC8482303.

50. Holmberg MJ, Granfeldt A, Mentzelopoulos SD, Andersen LW. Vasopressin and glucocorticoids for in-hospital cardiac arrest: A systematic review and meta-analysis of individual participant data. Resuscitation. 2022 Feb;171:48-56. doi: 10.1016/j.resuscitation.2021.12.030. Epub 2022 Jan 3. Erratum in: Resuscitation. 2023 Sep;190:109929. PMID: 34990764.

51. Bauer SR, Sacha GL, Lam SW, Wang L, Reddy AJ, Duggal A, Vachharajani V. Hemodynamic Response to Vasopressin Dosage of 0.03 Units/Min vs. 0.04 Units/Min in Patients With Septic Shock. J Intensive Care Med. 2022 Jan;37(1):92-99. doi: 10.1177/0885066620977181. Epub 2020 Nov 28. PMID: 33251906; PMCID: PMC10243460.

52. Lauzier F, Lévy B, Lamarre P, Lesur O. Vasopressin or norepinephrine in early hyperdynamic septic shock: a randomized clinical trial. Intensive Care Med. 2006 Nov;32(11):1782-9. doi: 10.1007/s00134-006-0378-0. Epub 2006 Sep 22. PMID: 17019548.

53. Hammond DA, Sacha GL, Bissell BD, et al: Effects of norepinephrine and vasopressin discontinuation order in the recovery phase of septic shock: A systematic review and individual patient data meta-analysis. Pharmacotherapy 2019; 39:544–552

54. Wu Z, Zhang S, Xu J, Xie J, Huang L, Huang Y, Yang Y, Qiu H. Norepinephrine vs Vasopressin: Which Vasopressor Should Be Discontinued First in Septic Shock? A Meta-Analysis. Shock. 2020 Jan;53(1):50-57. doi: 10.1097/ SHK.0000000000001345. PMID: 31008869.

55. Lam SW, Sacha GL, Duggal A, Reddy AJ, Bauer SR. Abrupt Discontinuation Versus Down-Titration of Vasopressin in Patients Recovering from Septic Shock. Shock. 2021 Feb 1;55(2):210-214. doi: 10.1097/ SHK.0000000000001609. PMID: 32842024.

56. Caldwell HK, Lee HJ, Macbeth AH, Young WS 3rd. Vasopressin: behavioral roles of an "original" neuropeptide. Prog Neurobiol. 2008 Jan;84(1):1-24. doi: 10.1016/j.pneurobio.2007.10.007. Epub 2007 Nov 4. PMID: 18053631; PMCID: PMC2292122.

57. Shampo MA, Kyle RA, Steensma DP. Stamp vignette on medical science. Vincent du Vigneaud-Nobel Prize in chemistry. Mayo Clin Proc. 2013 Sep;88(9):e99. doi: 10.1016/j.mayocp.2012.01.032. PMID: 24001505.

58. Glavaš M, Gitlin-Domagalska A, Dębowski D, Ptaszyńska N, Łęgowska A, Rolka K. Vasopressin and Its Analogues: From Natural Hormones to Multitasking Peptides. Int J Mol Sci. 2022 Mar 12;23(6):3068. doi: 10.3390/ ijms23063068. PMID: 35328489; PMCID: PMC8955888.

59. Bendicksen L, Kesselheim AS, Rome BN. The Vexing Voyage of Vasopressin: The Consequences of Granting Market Exclusivity to Unapproved Drugs. Chest. 2022 Aug;162(2):433-435. doi: 10.1016/j.chest.2022.02.048. PMID: 35940656; PMCID: PMC9353103.

60. Russell JA, Fjell C, Hsu JL, Lee T, Boyd J, Thair S, Singer J, Patterson AJ, Walley KR. Vasopressin compared with norepinephrine augments the decline of plasma cytokine levels in septic shock. Am J Respir Crit Care Med. 2013 Aug 1;188(3):356-64. doi: 10.1164/rccm.201302-0355OC. PMID: 23796235.

TERLIPRESSIN

. Bernadich C, Bandi JC, Melin P, Bosch J. Effects of F-180, a new selective vasoconstrictor peptide, compared with Terlipressin and vasopressin on systemic and splanchnic hemodynamics in a rat model of portal hypertension. Hepatology 1998;27:351–356. DOI: 10.1002/hep.510270206.

2. Demiselle J, Fage N, Radermacher P, Asfar P. Vasopressin and its analogues in shock states: a review. Ann Intensive Care 2020;10(1):9. doi: 10.1186/s13613-020-0628-2

3. "TERLIVAZ/Terlipressin Injection, USP." FDA.gov, U.S. Food and Drug Administration, 2023, https://www.accessdata.fda.gov/drugsatfda_docs/label/2022/022231s000lbl.pdf

4. Mårtensson J, Gordon AC. Terlipressin or norepinephrine, or both in septic shock? Intensive Care Med. 2018 Nov;44(11):1964-1966. doi: 10.1007/s00134-018-5290-x. Epub 2018 Jul 13. PMID: 30006892.

5. Jozwiak M. Alternatives to norepinephrine in septic shock: Which agents and when? J Intensive Med. 2022 Jun 12;2(4):223-232. doi: 10.1016/j.jointm.2022.05.001. PMID: 36788938; PMCID: PMC9924015.

6. Russell JA, Gordon AC, Williams MD, Boyd JH, Walley KR, Kissoon N. Vasopressor Therapy in the Intensive Care Unit. Semin Respir Crit Care Med. 2021 Feb;42(1):59-77. doi: 10.1055/s-0040-1710320. Epub 2020 Aug 20. PMID: 32820475.

7. Leone M, Albanèse J, Delmas A, Chaabane W, Garnier F, Martin C. Terlipressin in catecholamine-resistant septic shock patients. Shock. 2004 Oct;22(4):314-9. doi: 10.1097/01.shk.0000136097.42048.bd. PMID: 15377885.

8. Morelli A, Ertmer C, Rehberg S, Lange M, Orecchioni A, Cecchini V, Bachetoni A, D'Alessandro M, Van Aken H, Pietropaoli P, Westphal M. Continuous terlipressin versus vasopressin infusion in septic shock (TERLIVAP): a randomized, controlled pilot study. Crit Care. 2009;13(4):R130. doi: 10.1186/cc7990. Epub 2009 Aug 10. PMID: 19664253; PMCID: PMC2750187.

9. Liu ZM, Chen J, Kou Q, Lin Q, Huang X, Tang Z, Kang Y, Li K, Zhou L, Song Q, Sun T, Zhao L, Wang X, He X, Wang C, Wu B, Lin J, Yuan S, Gu Q, Qian K, Shi X, Feng Y, Lin A, He X; Study Group of investigators; Guan XD. Terlipressin versus norepinephrine as infusion in patients with septic shock: a multicentre, randomised, double-blinded trial. Intensive Care Med. 2018 Nov;44(11):1816-1825. doi: 10.1007/s00134-018-5267-9. Epub 2018 Jul 3. PMID: 29971593.

10. Sahoo P, Kothari N, Goyal S, Sharma A, Bhatia PK. Comparison of Norepinephrine and Terlipressin vs Norepinephrine Alone for Management of Septic Shock: A Randomized Control Study. Indian J Crit Care Med. 2022 Jun;26(6):669-675. doi: 10.5005/jp-journals-10071-24231. PMID: 35836627; PMCID: PMC9237141.

11. Evans L, Rhodes A, Alhazzani W, Antonelli M, Coopersmith CM, French C, Machado FR, Mcintyre L, Ostermann M, Prescott HC, Schorr C, Simpson S, Wiersinga WJ, Alshamsi F, Angus DC, Arabi Y, Azevedo L, Beale R, Beilman G, Belley-Cote E, Burry L, Cecconi M, Centofanti J, Coz Yataco A, De Waele J, Dellinger RP, Doi K, Du B, Estenssoro E, Ferrer R, Gomersall C, Hodgson C, Møller MH, Iwashyna T, Jacob S, Kleinpell R, Klompas M, Koh Y, Kumar A, Kwizera A, Lobo S, Masur H, McGloughlin S, Mehta S, Mehta Y, Mer M, Nunnally M, Oczkowski S, Osborn T, Papathanassoglou E, Perner A, Puskarich M, Roberts J, Schweickert W, Seckel M, Sevransky J, Sprung CL, Welte T, Zimmerman J, Levy M. Surviving sepsis campaign: international guidelines for management of sepsis and septic shock 2021. Intensive Care Med. 2021 Nov;47(11):1181-1247. doi: 10.1007/s00134-021-06506-y. Epub 2021 Oct 2. PMID: 34599691; PMCID: PMC8486643.

12. Zhu Y, Huang H, Xi X, Du B. Terlipressin for septic shock patients: a meta-analysis of randomized controlled study. J Intensive Care. 2019 Mar 12;7:16. doi: 10.1186/s40560-019-0369-1. PMID: 30923620; PMCID: PMC6419496.

13. Huang L, Zhang S, Chang W, Xia F, Liu S, Yang Y, Qiu H. Terlipressin for the treatment of septic shock in adults: a systematic review and meta-analysis. BMC Anesthesiol. 2020 Mar 5;20(1):58. doi: 10.1186/s12871-020-00965-4. PMID: 32138657; PMCID: PMC7057452.

14. Williams MD, Russell JA. Terlipressin or norepinephrine in septic shock: do we have the answer? J Thorac Dis. 2019 May;11(Suppl 9):S1270-S1273. doi: 10.21037/jtd.2019.05.07. PMID: 31245106; PMCID: PMC6560608.

15. Yao RQ, Xia DM, Wang LX, Wu GS, Zhu YB, Zhao HQ, Liu Q, Xia ZF, Ren C, Yao YM. Clinical Efficiency of Vasopressin or Its Analogs in Comparison With Catecholamines Alone on Patients With Septic Shock: A Systematic Review and Meta-Analysis. Front Pharmacol. 2020 May 6;11:563. doi: 10.3389/fphar.2020.00563. PMID: 32435192; PMCID: PMC7218087.

16. Wang J, Shi M, Huang L, Li Q, Meng S, Xu J, Xue M, Xie J, Liu S, Huang Y. Addition of terlipressin to norepinephrine in septic shock and effect of renal perfusion: a pilot study. Ren Fail. 2022 Dec;44(1):1207-1215. doi: 10.1080/0886022X.2022.2095286. PMID: 35856162; PMCID: PMC9307113.

17. Schultz J, Andersen A, Lyhne MD, Arcanjo DDR, Kjaergaard B, Simonsen U, Nielsen-Kudsk JE. Terlipressin Increases Systemic and Lowers Pulmonary Arterial Pressure in Experimental Acute Pulmonary Embolism. Crit Care Med. 2020 Apr;48(4):e308-e315. doi: 10.1097/CCM.0000000000004243. PMID: 32205621.

18. Levy B, Fritz C, Tahon E, Jacquot A, Auchet T, Kimmoun A. Vasoplegia treatments: the past, the present, and the future. Crit Care. 2018 Feb 27;22(1):52. doi: 10.1186/s13054-018-1967-3. PMID: 29486781; PMCID: PMC6389278.

19. Subedi A, Suresh Kumar VC, Sharma Subedi A, Sapkota B. A Review of Hepatorenal Syndrome. Cureus. 2021 Jul 1;13(7):e16084. doi: 10.7759/cureus.16084. PMID: 34367745; PMCID: PMC8330394.

20. Wang H, Liu A, Bo W, Feng X, Hu Y. Terlipressin in the treatment of hepatorenal syndrome: A systematic review and meta-analysis. Medicine (Baltimore). 2018 Apr;97(16):e0431. doi: 10.1097/MD.0000000000010431. PMID: 29668606; PMCID: PMC5916651.

21. European Association for the Study of the Liver. Electronic address: easloffice@easloffice.eu; European Association for the Study of the Liver. EASL Clinical Practice Guidelines for the management of patients with decompensated cirrhosis. J Hepatol. 2018 Aug;69(2):406-460. doi: 10.1016/j.jhep.2018.03.024. Epub 2018 Apr 10. Erratum in: J Hepatol. 2018 Nov;69(5):1207. PMID: 29653741.

22. Wong F, Pappas SC, Curry MP, Reddy KR, Rubin RA, Porayko MK, Gonzalez SA, Mumtaz K, Lim N, Simonetto DA, Sharma P, Sanyal AJ, Mayo MJ, Frederick RT, Escalante S, Jamil K; CONFIRM Study Investigators. Terlipressin plus Albumin for the Treatment of Type 1 Hepatorenal Syndrome. N Engl J Med. 2021 Mar 4;384(9):818-828. doi: 10.1056/NEJMoa2008290. PMID: 33657294.

SELEPRESSIN
1. Lövgren U, Johansson S, Jensen LS, Ekström C, Carlshaf A. Quantitative determination of peptide drug in human plasma samples at low pg/ml levels using coupled column liquid chromatography-tandem mass spectrometry. J Pharm Biomed Anal. 2010 Nov 2;53(3):537-45. doi: 10.1016/j.jpba.2010.03.024. Epub 2010 Mar 27. PMID: 20456896.
2. Rehberg S, Ertmer C, Vincent JL, Morelli A, Schneider M, Lange M, Van Aken H, Traber DL, Westphal M. Role of selective V1a receptor agonism in ovine septic shock. Crit Care Med. 2011 Jan;39(1):119-25. doi: 10.1097/CCM.0b013e3181fa3898. PMID: 20890184.
3. Rehberg S, Yamamoto Y, Sousse L, Bartha E, Jonkam C, Hasselbach AK, Traber LD, Cox RA, Westphal M, Enkhbaatar P, Traber DL. Selective V(1a) agonism attenuates vascular dysfunction and fluid accumulation in ovine severe sepsis. Am J Physiol Heart Circ Physiol. 2012 Nov 15;303(10):H1245-54. doi: 10.1152/ajpheart.00390.2012. Epub 2012 Sep 7. PMID: 22961865; PMCID: PMC3517638.
4. Maybauer MO, Maybauer DM, Enkhbaatar P, Laporte R, Wiśniewska H, Traber LD, Lin C, Fan J, Hawkins HK, Cox RA, Wiśniewski K, Schteingart CD, Landry DW, Rivière PJ, Traber DL. Selective vasopressin type 1a receptor agonist selepressin (FE 202158) blocks vascular leak in ovine severe sepsis*. Crit Care Med. 2014 Jul;42(7):e525-e533. doi: 10.1097/CCM.0000000000000300. PMID: 24674922; PMCID: PMC4346299.
5. He X, Su F, Taccone FS, Laporte R, Kjølbye AL, Zhang J, Xie K, Moussa MD, Reinheimer TM, Vincent JL. A Selective V(1A) Receptor Agonist, Selepressin, Is Superior to Arginine Vasopressin and to Norepinephrine in Ovine Septic Shock. Crit Care Med. 2016 Jan;44(1):23-31. doi: 10.1097/CCM.0000000000001380. PMID: 26496451; PMCID: PMC4684247.
6. Barabutis N, Marinova M, Solopov P, Uddin MA, Croston GE, Reinheimer TM, Catravas JD. Protective Mechanism of the Selective Vasopressin V1A Receptor Agonist Selepressin against Endothelial Barrier Dysfunction. J Pharmacol Exp Ther. 2020 Nov;375(2):286-295. doi: 10.1124/jpet.120.000146. Epub 2020 Sep 17. PMID: 32943478.
7. Milano SP, Boucheix OB, Reinheimer TM. Selepressin, a novel selective V1A receptor agonist: Effect on mesenteric flow and gastric mucosa perfusion in the endotoxemic rabbit. Peptides. 2020 Jul;129:170318. doi: 10.1016/j.peptides.2020.170318. Epub 2020 Apr 22. PMID: 32330539.
8. Russell JA, Vincent JL, Kjølbye AL, Olsson H, Blemings A, Spapen H, Carl P, Laterre PF, Grundemar L. Selepressin, a novel selective vasopressin V1A agonist, is an effective substitute for norepinephrine in a phase IIa randomized, placebo-controlled trial in septic shock patients. Crit Care. 2017 Aug 15;21(1):213. doi: 10.1186/s13054-017-1798-7. PMID: 28807037; PMCID: PMC5557574.
9. Laterre PF, Berry SM, Blemings A, Carlsen JE, François B, Graves T, Jacobsen K, Lewis RJ, Opal SM, Perner A, Pickkers P, Russell JA, Windeløv NA, Yealy DM, Asfar P, Bestle MH, Muller G, Bruel C, Brulé N, Decruyenaere J, Dive AM, Dugernier T, Krell K, Lefrant JY, Megarbane B, Mercier E, Mira JP, Quenot JP, Rasmussen BS, Thorsen-Meyer HC, Vander Laenen M, Vang ML, Vignon P, Vinatier I, Wichmann S, Wittebole X, Kjølbye AL, Angus DC; SEPSIS-ACT Investigators. Effect of Selepressin vs Placebo on Ventilator- and Vasopressor-Free Days in Patients With Septic Shock: The SEPSIS-ACT Randomized Clinical Trial. JAMA. 2019 Oct 15;322(15):1476-1485. doi: 10.1001/jama.2019.14607. Erratum in: JAMA. 2019 Nov 12;322(18):1830. PMID: 31577035; PMCID: PMC6802260.
10. Marks JA, Pascual JL. Selepressin in septic shock: sharpening the VASST effects of vasopressin?*. Crit Care Med. 2014 Jul;42(7):1747-8. doi: 10.1097/CCM.0000000000000420. PMID: 24933060.
11. Levy B, Fritz C, Tahon E, Jacquot A, Auchet T, Kimmoun A. Vasoplegia treatments: the past, the present, and the future. Crit Care. 2018 Feb 27;22(1):52. doi: 10.1186/s13054-018-1967-3. PMID: 29486781; PMCID: PMC6389278.
12. Stolk RF, van der Poll T, Angus DC, van der Hoeven JG, Pickkers P, Kox M. Potentially Inadvertent Immunomodulation: Norepinephrine Use in Sepsis. Am J Respir Crit Care Med. 2016 Sep 1;194(5):550-8. doi: 10.1164/rccm.201604-0862CP. PMID: 27398737.
13. Hajjar LA, Vincent JL, Barbosa Gomes Galas FR, Rhodes A, Landoni G, Osawa EA, Melo RR, Sundin MR, Grande SM, Gaiotto FA, Pomerantzeff PM, Dallan LO, Franco RA, Nakamura RE, Lisboa LA, de Almeida JP, Gerent AM, Souza DH, Gaiane MA, Fukushima JT, Park CL, Zambolim C, Rocha Ferreira GS, Strabelli TM, Fernandes FL, Camara L, Zeferino S, Santos VG, Piccioni MA, Jatene FB, Costa Auler JO Jr, Filho RK. Vasopressin versus Norepinephrine in Patients with Vasoplegic Shock after Cardiac Surgery: The VANCS Randomized Controlled Trial. Anesthesiology. 2017 Jan;126(1):85-93. doi: 10.1097/ALN.0000000000001434. PMID: 27841822.

DOPAMINE
1. Triposkiadis FK, Butler J, Karayannis G, Starling RC, Filippatos G, Wolski K, Parissis J, Parisis C, Rovithis D, Koutrakis K, Skoularigis J, Antoniou CK, Chrysohoou C, Pitsavos C, Stefanadis C, Nastas J, Tsaknakis T, Mantziari L, Giannakoulas G, Karvounis H, Kalogeropoulos AP, Giamouzis G. Efficacy and safety of high dose versus low dose furosemide with or without dopamine infusion: the Dopamine in Acute Decompensated Heart Failure II (DAD-HF II) trial. Int J Cardiol. 2014 Mar 1;172(1):115-21. doi: 10.1016/j.ijcard.2013.12.276. Epub 2014 Jan 10. PMID: 24485633.
2. Chen HH, Anstrom KJ, Givertz MM, Stevenson LW, Semigran MJ, Goldsmith SR, Bart BA, Bull DA, Stehlik J, LeWinter MM, Konstam MA, Huggins GS, Rouleau JL, O'Meara E, Tang WH, Starling RC, Butler J, Deswal A, Felker GM, O'Connor CM, Bonita RE, Margulies KB, Cappola TP, Ofili EO, Mann DL, Dávila-Román VG, McNulty SE, Borlaug BA, Velazquez EJ, Lee KL, Shah MR, Hernandez AF, Braunwald E, Redfield MM; NHLBI Heart Failure Clinical Research Network. Low-dose dopamine or low-dose nesiritide in acute heart failure with renal dysfunction: the ROSE acute heart failure randomized trial. JAMA. 2013 Dec 18;310(23):2533-43. doi: 10.1001/jama.2013.282190. PMID: 24247300; PMCID: PMC3934929.

3. Russell JA, Gordon AC, Williams MD, Boyd JH, Walley KR, Kissoon N. Vasopressor Therapy in the Intensive Care Unit. Semin Respir Crit Care Med. 2021 Feb;42(1):59-77. doi: 10.1055/s-0040-1710320. Epub 2020 Aug 20. PMID: 32820475.
4. Dopamine Package Insert
5. Hollenberg SM. Vasopressor support in septic shock. Chest. 2007 Nov;132(5):1678-87. doi: 10.1378/chest.07-0291. PMID: 17998371.
6. Jozwiak M. Alternatives to norepinephrine in septic shock: Which agents and when? J Intensive Med. 2022 Jun 12;2(4):223-232. doi: 10.1016/j.jointm.2022.05.001. PMID: 36788938; PMCID: PMC9924015.
7. Overgaard CB, Dzavík V. Inotropes and vasopressors: review of physiology and clinical use in cardiovascular disease. Circulation. 2008 Sep 2;118(10):1047-56. doi: 10.1161/CIRCULATIONAHA.107.728840. PMID: 18765387.
8. Bangash MN, Kong ML, Pearse RM. Use of inotropes and vasopressor agents in critically ill patients. Br J Pharmacol. 2012 Apr;165(7):2015-33. doi: 10.1111/j.1476-5381.2011.01588.x. PMID: 21740415; PMCID: PMC3413841.
9. Debaveye YA, Van den Berghe GH. Is there still a place for dopamine in the modern intensive care unit? Anesth Analg. 2004 Feb;98(2):461-468. doi: 10.1213/01.ANE.0000096188.35789.37. PMID: 14742388.
10. Juste RN, Moran L, Hooper J, Soni N. Dopamine clearance in critically ill patients. Intensive Care Med. 1998 Nov;24(11):1217-20. doi: 10.1007/s001340050747. PMID: 9876986.
11. De Backer D, Aldecoa C, Njimi H, Vincent JL. Dopamine versus norepinephrine in the treatment of septic shock: a meta-analysis*. Crit Care Med. 2012 Mar;40(3):725-30. doi: 10.1097/CCM.0b013e31823778ee. PMID: 22036860.
12. Dellinger RP, Levy MM, Rhodes A, Annane D, Gerlach H, Opal SM, Sevransky JE, Sprung CL, Douglas IS, Jaeschke R, Osborn TM, Nunnally ME, Townsend SR, Reinhart K, Kleinpell RM, Angus DC, Deutschman CS, Machado FR, Rubenfeld GD, Webb SA, Beale RJ, Vincent JL, Moreno R; Surviving Sepsis Campaign Guidelines Committee including the Pediatric Subgroup. Surviving sepsis campaign: international guidelines for management of severe sepsis and septic shock: 2012. Crit Care Med. 2013 Feb;41(2):580-637. doi: 10.1097/CCM.0b013e31827e83af. PMID: 23353941.
13. Evans L, Rhodes A, Alhazzani W, Antonelli M, Coopersmith CM, French C, Machado FR, Mcintyre L, Ostermann M, Prescott HC, Schorr C, Simpson S, Wiersinga WJ, Alshamsi F, Angus DC, Arabi Y, Azevedo L, Beale R, Beilman G, Belley-Cote E, Burry L, Cecconi M, Centofanti J, Coz Yataco A, De Waele J, Dellinger RP, Doi K, Du B, Estenssoro E, Ferrer R, Gomersall C, Hodgson C, Møller MH, Iwashyna T, Jacob S, Kleinpell R, Klompas M, Koh Y, Kumar A, Kwizera A, Lobo S, Masur H, McGloughlin S, Mehta S, Mehta Y, Mer M, Nunnally M, Oczkowski S, Osborn T, Papathanassoglou E, Perner A, Puskarich M, Roberts J, Schweickert W, Seckel M, Sevransky J, Sprung CL, Welte T, Zimmerman J, Levy M. Surviving sepsis campaign: international guidelines for management of sepsis and septic shock 2021. Intensive Care Med. 2021 Nov;47(11):1181-1247. doi: 10.1007/s00134-021-06506-y. Epub 2021 Oct 2. PMID: 34599691; PMCID: PMC8486643.
14. Rui Q, Jiang Y, Chen M, Zhang N, Yang H, Zhou Y. Dopamine versus norepinephrine in the treatment of cardiogenic shock: A PRISMA-compliant meta-analysis. Medicine (Baltimore). 2017 Oct;96(43):e8402. doi: 10.1097/MD.0000000000008402. PMID: 29069037; PMCID: PMC5671870.
15. Ponikowski P, Voors AA, Anker SD, Bueno H, Cleland JGF, Coats AJS, Falk V, González-Juanatey JR, Harjola VP, Jankowska EA, Jessup M, Linde C, Nihoyannopoulos P, Parissis JT, Pieske B, Riley JP, Rosano GMC, Ruilope LM, Ruschitzka F, Rutten FH, van der Meer P; ESC Scientific Document Group. 2016 ESC Guidelines for the diagnosis and treatment of acute and chronic heart failure: The Task Force for the diagnosis and treatment of acute and chronic heart failure of the European Society of Cardiology (ESC)Developed with the special contribution of the Heart Failure Association (HFA) of the ESC. Eur Heart J. 2016 Jul 14;37(27):2129-2200. doi: 10.1093/eurheartj/ehw128. Epub 2016 May 20. Erratum in: Eur Heart J. 2016 Dec 30;: PMID: 27206819.
16. van Diepen S, Katz JN, Albert NM, Henry TD, Jacobs AK, Kapur NK, Kilic A, Menon V, Ohman EM, Sweitzer NK, Thiele H, Washam JB, Cohen MG; American Heart Association Council on Clinical Cardiology; Council on Cardiovascular and Stroke Nursing; Council on Quality of Care and Outcomes Research; and Mission: Lifeline. Contemporary Management of Cardiogenic Shock: A Scientific Statement From the American Heart Association. Circulation. 2017 Oct 17;136(16):e232-e268. doi: 10.1161/CIR.0000000000000525. Epub 2017 Sep 18. PMID: 28923988.
17. Bellomo R, Chapman M, Finfer S, Hickling K, Myburgh J. Low-dose dopamine in patients with early renal dysfunction: a placebo-controlled randomised trial. Australian and New Zealand Intensive Care Society (ANZICS) Clinical Trials Group. Lancet. 2000 Dec 23-30;356(9248):2139-43. doi: 10.1016/s0140-6736(00)03495-4. PMID: 11191541.
18. Joannidis M, Druml W, Forni LG, Groeneveld ABJ, Honore PM, Hoste E, Ostermann M, Oudemans-van Straaten HM, Schetz M. Prevention of acute kidney injury and protection of renal function in the intensive care unit: update 2017 : Expert opinion of the Working Group on Prevention, AKI section, European Society of Intensive Care Medicine. Intensive Care Med. 2017 Jun;43(6):730-749. doi: 10.1007/s00134-017-4832-y. Epub 2017 Jun 2. PMID: 28577069; PMCID: PMC5487598.
19. Schnuelle P, Gottmann U, Hoeger S, Boesebeck D, Lauchart W, Weiss C, Fischereder M, Jauch KW, Heemann U, Zeier M, Hugo C, Pisarski P, Krämer BK, Lopau K, Rahmel A, Benck U, Birck R, Yard BA. Effects of donor pretreatment with dopamine on graft function after kidney transplantation: a randomized controlled trial. JAMA. 2009 Sep 9;302(10):1067-75. doi: 10.1001/jama.2009.1310. PMID: 19738091.
20. Hollenberg SM. Vasopressor support in septic shock. Chest. 2007 Nov;132(5):1678-87. doi: 10.1378/chest.07-0291. PMID: 17998371.

21. Beck GCh, Brinkkoetter P, Hanusch C, Schulte J, van Ackern K, van der Woude FJ, Yard BA. Clinical review: immunomodulatory effects of dopamine in general inflammation. Crit Care. 2004 Dec;8(6):485-91. doi: 10.1186/cc2879. Epub 2004 Jun 3. PMID: 15566620; PMCID: PMC1065039.
22. Galley HF. Renal-dose dopamine: will the message now get through? Lancet. 2000 Dec 23-30;356(9248):2112-3. doi: 10.1016/S0140-6736(00)03484-X. Erratum in: Lancet 2001 Mar 17;357(9259):890. PMID: 11191531.
23. Holmes CL, Walley KR. Bad medicine: low-dose dopamine in the ICU. Chest. 2003 Apr;123(4):1266-75. doi: 10.1378/chest.123.4.1266. PMID: 12684320.
24. Marinosci GZ, De Robertis E, De Benedictis G, Piazza O. Dopamine Use in Intensive Care: Are We Ready to Turn it Down? Transl Med UniSa. 2012 Oct 11;4:90-4. PMID: 23905068; PMCID: PMC3728808.
25. GOLDBERG LI, MCDONALD RH Jr, ZIMMERMAN AM. SODIUM DIURESIS PRODUCED BY DOPAMINE IN PATIENTS WITH CONGESTIVE HEART FAILURE. N Engl J Med. 1963 Nov 14;269:1060-4. doi: 10.1056/NEJM196311142692003. PMID: 14085064.
26. Kellum JA, M Decker J. Use of dopamine in acute renal failure: a meta-analysis. Crit Care Med. 2001 Aug;29(8):1526-31. doi: 10.1097/00003246-200108000-00005. PMID: 11505120.
27. Marik PE. Low-dose dopamine: a systematic review. Intensive Care Med. 2002 Jul;28(7):877-83. doi: 10.1007/s00134-002-1346-y. Epub 2002 May 31. PMID: 12122525.
28. Schnuelle P, Yard BA, Braun C, Dominguez-Fernandez E, Schaub M, Birck R, Sturm J, Post S, van der Woude FJ. Impact of donor dopamine on immediate graft function after kidney transplantation. Am J Transplant. 2004 Mar;4(3):419-26. doi: 10.1111/j.1600-6143.2004.00331.x. PMID: 14961996.
29. Kotloff RM, Blosser S, Fulda GJ, Malinoski D, Ahya VN, Angel L, Byrnes MC, DeVita MA, Grissom TE, Halpern SD, Nakagawa TA, Stock PG, Sudan DL, Wood KE, Anillo SJ, Bleck TP, Eidbo EE, Fowler RA, Glazier AK, Gries C, Hasz R, Herr D, Khan A, Landsberg D, Lebovitz DJ, Levine DJ, Mathur M, Naik P, Niemann CU, Nunley DR, O'Connor KJ, Pelletier SJ, Rahman O, Ranjan D, Salim A, Sawyer RG, Shafer T, Sonneti D, Spiro P, Valapour M, Vikraman-Sushama D, Whelan TP; Society of Critical Care Medicine/American College of Chest Physicians/Association of Organ Procurement Organizations Donor Management Task Force. Management of the Potential Organ Donor in the ICU: Society of Critical Care Medicine/American College of Chest Physicians/Association of Organ Procurement Organizations Consensus Statement. Crit Care Med. 2015 Jun;43(6):1291-325. doi: 10.1097/CCM.0000000000000958. PMID: 25978154.

ANGIOTENSIN II

1. Khanna A, English SW, Wang XS, Ham K, Tumlin J, Szerlip H, Busse LW, Altaweel L, Albertson TE, Mackey C, McCurdy MT, Boldt DW, Chock S, Young PJ, Krell K, Wunderink RG, Ostermann M, Murugan R, Gong MN, Panwar R, Hästbacka J, Favory R, Venkatesh B, Thompson BT, Bellomo R, Jensen J, Kroll S, Chawla LS, Tidmarsh GF, Deane AM; ATHOS-3 Investigators. Angiotensin II for the Treatment of Vasodilatory Shock. N Engl J Med. 2017 Aug 3;377(5):419-430. doi: 10.1056/NEJMoa1704154. Epub 2017 May 21. PMID: 28528561.
2. GIAPREZA (angiotensin II) Injection for Intravenous Infusion. Initial U.S. Approval: 2017 Manufactured for: La Jolla Pharmaceutical Company. San Diego, CA 92121. Revised: 1/2018
3. Buchtele N, Schwameis M, Jilma B. Angiotensin II for the treatment of vasodilatory shock: enough data to consider angiotensin II safe? Crit Care. 2018 Apr 16;22(1):96. doi: 10.1186/s13054-018-2006-0. PMID: 29661216; PMCID: PMC5902841.
4. Wieruszewski PM, Wittwer ED, Kashani KB, Brown DR, Butler SO, Clark AM, Cooper CJ, Davison DL, Gajic O, Gunnerson KJ, Tendler R, Mara KC, Barreto EF. Angiotensin II Infusion for Shock: A Multicenter Study of Postmarketing Use. Chest. 2021 Feb;159(2):596-605. doi: 10.1016/j.chest.2020.08.2074. Epub 2020 Aug 31. PMID: 32882250; PMCID: PMC7856533.
5. Smith SE, Newsome AS, Guo Y, Hecht J, McCurdy MT, Mazzeffi MA, Chow JH, Kethireddy S. A Multicenter Observational Cohort Study of Angiotensin II in Shock. J Intensive Care Med. 2022 Jan;37(1):75-82. doi: 10.1177/0885066620972943. Epub 2020 Nov 24. PMID: 33231111; PMCID: PMC8559525.
6. Bellomo R, Wunderink RG, Szerlip H, English SW, Busse LW, Deane AM, Khanna AK, McCurdy MT, Ostermann M, Young PJ, Handisides DR, Chawla LS, Tidmarsh GF, Albertson TE. Angiotensin I and angiotensin II concentrations and their ratio in catecholamine-resistant vasodilatory shock. Crit Care. 2020 Feb 6;24(1):43. doi: 10.1186/s13054-020-2733-x. PMID: 32028998; PMCID: PMC7006163.
7. Bellomo R, Forni LG, Busse LW, McCurdy MT, Ham KR, Boldt DW, Hästbacka J, Khanna AK, Albertson TE, Tumlin J, Storey K, Handisides D, Tidmarsh GF, Chawla LS, Ostermann M. Renin and Survival in Patients Given Angiotensin II for Catecholamine-Resistant Vasodilatory Shock. A Clinical Trial. Am J Respir Crit Care Med. 2020 Nov 1;202(9):1253-1261. doi: 10.1164/rccm.201911-2172OC. PMID: 32609011; PMCID: PMC7605187.
8. Chow JH, Wittwer ED, Wieruszewski PM, Khanna AK. Evaluating the evidence for angiotensin II for the treatment of vasoplegia in critically ill cardiothoracic surgery patients. J Thorac Cardiovasc Surg. 2022 Apr;163(4):1407-1414. doi: 10.1016/j.jtcvs.2021.02.097. Epub 2021 Mar 19. PMID: 33875258.
9. Wieruszewski PM, Bellomo R, Busse LW, Ham KR, Zarbock A, Khanna AK, Deane AM, Ostermann M, Wunderink RG, Boldt DW, Kroll S, Greenfeld CR, Hodges T, Chow JH; Angiotensin II for the Treatment of High-Output Shock 3 (ATHOS-3) Investigators. Initiating angiotensin II at lower vasopressor doses in vasodilatory shock: an exploratory post-hoc analysis of the ATHOS-3 clinical trial. Crit Care. 2023 May 5;27(1):175. doi: 10.1186/s13054-023-04446-1. PMID: 37147690; PMCID: PMC10163684.
10. Quan M, Cho N, Bushell T, Mak J, Nguyen N, Litwak J, Rockwood N, Nguyen HB. Effectiveness of Angiotensin II for Catecholamine Refractory Septic or Distributive Shock on Mortality: A Propensity Score Weighted Analysis of Real-World Experience in the Medical ICU. Crit Care Explor. 2022 Jan 18;4(1):e0623. doi: 10.1097/CCE.0000000000000623. PMID: 35072084; PMCID: PMC8769135.

11. Russell JA, Walley KR, Singer J, Gordon AC, Hébert PC, Cooper DJ, Holmes CL, Mehta S, Granton JT, Storms MM, Cook DJ, Presneill JJ, Ayers D; VASST Investigators. Vasopressin versus norepinephrine infusion in patients with septic shock. N Engl J Med. 2008 Feb 28;358(9):877-87. doi: 10.1056/NEJMoa067373. PMID: 18305265.
12. Gordon AC, Mason AJ, Thirunavukkarasu N, Perkins GD, Cecconi M, Cepkova M, Pogson DG, Aya HD, Anjum A, Frazier GJ, Santhakumaran S, Ashby D, Brett SJ; VANISH Investigators. Effect of Early Vasopressin vs Norepinephrine on Kidney Failure in Patients With Septic Shock: The VANISH Randomized Clinical Trial. JAMA. 2016 Aug 2;316(5):509-18. doi: 10.1001/jama.2016.10485. PMID: 27483065.
13. Tumlin JA, Murugan R, Deane AM, Ostermann M, Busse LW, Ham KR, Kashani K, Szerlip HM, Prowle JR, Bihorac A, Finkel KW, Zarbock A, Forni LG, Lynch SJ, Jensen J, Kroll S, Chawla LS, Tidmarsh GF, Bellomo R; Angiotensin II for the Treatment of High-Output Shock 3 (ATHOS-3) Investigators. Outcomes in Patients with Vasodilatory Shock and Renal Replacement Therapy Treated with Intravenous Angiotensin II. Crit Care Med. 2018 Jun;46(6):949-957. doi: 10.1097/CCM.0000000000003092. Erratum in: Crit Care Med. 2018 Aug;46(8):e824. PMID: 29509568; PMCID: PMC5959265.
14. See EJ, Clapham C, Liu J, Khasin M, Liskaser G, Chan JW, Serpa Neto A, Costa Pinto R, Bellomo R. A PILOT STUDY OF ANGIOTENSIN II AS PRIMARY VASOPRESSOR IN CRITICALLY ILL ADULTS WITH VASODILATORY HYPOTENSION: THE ARAMIS STUDY. Shock. 2023 May 1;59(5):691-696. doi: 10.1097/SHK.0000000000002109. Epub 2023 Mar 18. PMID: 36930693.
15. Klijian A, Khanna AK, Reddy VS, Friedman B, Ortoleva J, Evans AS, Panwar R, Kroll S, Greenfeld CR, Chatterjee S. Treatment With Angiotensin II Is Associated With Rapid Blood Pressure Response and Vasopressor Sparing in Patients With Vasoplegia After Cardiac Surgery: A Post-Hoc Analysis of Angiotensin II for the Treatment of High-Output Shock (ATHOS-3) Study. J Cardiothorac Vasc Anesth. 2021 Jan;35(1):51-58. doi: 10.1053/j.jvca.2020.08.001. Epub 2020 Aug 7. PMID: 32868152.
16. Coulson TG, Miles LF, Serpa Neto A, Pilcher D, Weinberg L, Landoni G, Zarbock A, Bellomo R. A double-blind, randomised feasibility trial of angiotensin-2 in cardiac surgery. Anaesthesia. 2022 Sep;77(9):999-1009. doi: 10.1111/anae.15802. PMID: 35915923; PMCID: PMC9543254.
17. Chow JH, Wittwer ED, Wieruszewski PM, Khanna AK. Evaluating the evidence for angiotensin II for the treatment of vasoplegia in critically ill cardiothoracic surgery patients. J Thorac Cardiovasc Surg. 2022 Apr;163(4):1407-1414. doi: 10.1016/j.jtcvs.2021.02.097. Epub 2021 Mar 19. PMID: 33875258.
18. WEDEEN R, ZUCKER G. Angiotensin II in the treatment of shock. Am J Cardiol. 1963 Jan;11:82-6. doi: 10.1016/0002-9149(63)90036-5. PMID: 13999441.
19. BEANLANDS DS, GUNTON RW. ANGIOTENSIN II IN THE TREATMENT OF SHOCK FOLLOWING MYOCARDIAL INFARCTION. Am J Cardiol. 1964 Sep;14:370-3. doi: 10.1016/0002-9149(64)90081-5. PMID: 14206184.
20. Busse LW, McCurdy MT, Ali O, Hall A, Chen H, Ostermann M. The effect of angiotensin II on blood pressure in patients with circulatory shock: a structured review of the literature. Crit Care. 2017 Dec 28;21(1):324. doi: 10.1186/s13054-017-1896-6. PMID: 29282149; PMCID: PMC5745607.
21. Wieruszewski PM, Seelhammer TG, Barreto EF, Busse LW, Chow JH, Davison DL, Gaglani B, Khanna AK, Ten Lohuis CC, Mara KC, Wittwer ED. Angiotensin II for Vasodilatory Hypotension in Patients Requiring Mechanical Circulatory Support. J Intensive Care Med. 2023 May;38(5):464-471. doi: 10.1177/08850666221145864. Epub 2022 Dec 15. PMID: 36524274.
22. Mohamed A, Berry TP, Welge JA, Thomas EL, Zhurav L, Kozinn J, Haines MM. Angiotensin II in Patients With Shock on Mechanical Circulatory Support: A Single-Center Retrospective Case Series. J Cardiothorac Vasc Anesth. 2022 Aug;36(8 Pt A):2439-2445. doi: 10.1053/j.jvca.2022.01.002. Epub 2022 Jan 7. PMID: 35144869.
23. Alam A, Sovic W, Gill J, Ragula N, Salem M, Hughes GJ, Colbert GB, Mooney JL. Angiotensin II: A Review of Current Literature. J Cardiothorac Vasc Anesth. 2022 Apr;36(4):1180-1187. doi: 10.1053/j.jvca.2021.07.021. Epub 2021 Jul 16. PMID: 34452817.
24. Antonucci E, Agosta S, Sakr Y. Angiotensin II in vasodilatory shock: lights and shadows. Crit Care. 2017 Nov 14;21(1):277. doi: 10.1186/s13054-017-1869-9. PMID: 29137677; PMCID: PMC5686834.
25. Page IH, Helmer OM. A CRYSTALLINE PRESSOR SUBSTANCE (ANGIOTONIN) RESULTING FROM THE REACTION BETWEEN RENIN AND RENIN-ACTIVATOR. J Exp Med. 1940 Jan 1;71(1):29-42. doi: 10.1084/jem.71.1.29. PMID: 19870942; PMCID: PMC2134997.
26. Knaus WA, Draper EA, Wagner DP, Zimmerman JE. APACHE II: a severity of disease classification system. Crit Care Med. 1985 Oct;13(10):818-29. PMID: 3928249.
27. Lipworth BJ, Dagg KD. Vasoconstrictor effects of angiotensin II on the pulmonary vascular bed. Chest. 1994 May;105(5):1360-4. doi: 10.1378/chest.105.5.1360. PMID: 8181320.
28. E. Braun Menendez et al. Angiotonin or Hypertensin. Science 98,495-495(1943). DOI:10.1126/science.98.2553.495.a
29. (2017, December 21). FDA approves drug to treat dangerously low blood pressure. FDA.gov. Retrieved November 6, 2023, from https://www.fda.gov/news-events/press-announcements/fda-approves-drug-treat-dangerously-low-blood-pressure

MIDODRINE

1. Midodrine [package insert]. Shire US Inc. 300 Shire Way, Lexington, MA 02421, USA. Accessed October 2, 2023. Available at: ProAmatine (midodrine hydrochloride) Label. fda.gov; 2023.
2. Zakir RM, Folefack A, Saric M, Berkowitz RL. The use of midodrine in patients with advanced heart failure. Congest Heart Fail. 2009 May-Jun;15(3):108-11. doi: 10.1111/j.1751-7133.2008.00042.x. PMID: 19522958.

3. Macielak SA, Vollmer NJ, Haddad NA, Nabzdyk CGS, Nei SD. Hemodynamic Effects of an Increased Midodrine Dosing Frequency. Crit Care Explor. 2021 Apr 26;3(4):e0405. doi: 10.1097/CCE.0000000000000405. PMID: 33912835; PMCID: PMC8078337.
4. Whitson MR, Mo E, Nabi T, Healy L, Koenig S, Narasimhan M, Mayo PH. Feasibility, Utility, and Safety of Midodrine During Recovery Phase From Septic Shock. Chest. 2016 Jun;149(6):1380-3. doi: 10.1016/j.chest.2016.02.657. Epub 2016 Mar 4. PMID: 26953217.
5. Hammond DA, Smith MN, Meena N. Considerations on Midodrine Use in Resolving Septic Shock. Chest. 2016 Jun;149(6):1582-3. doi: 10.1016/j.chest.2016.03.054. PMID: 27287581.
6. Hammond DA, Smith MN, Peksa GD, Trivedi AP, Balk RA, Menich BE. Midodrine as an Adjuvant to Intravenous Vasopressor Agents in Adults With Resolving Shock: Systematic Review and Meta-Analysis. J Intensive Care Med. 2020 Nov;35(11):1209-1215. doi: 10.1177/0885066619843279. Epub 2019 Apr 28. PMID: 31030630.
7. Rizvi MS, Trivedi V, Nasim F, Lin E, Kashyap R, Andrijasevic N, Gajic O. Trends in Use of Midodrine in the ICU: A Single-Center Retrospective Case Series. Crit Care Med. 2018 Jul;46(7):e628-e633. doi: 10.1097/CCM.0000000000003121. PMID: 29613861.
8. Levine AR, Meyer MJ, Bittner EA, Berg S, Kalman R, Stanislaus AB, Ryan C, Ball SA, Eikermann M. Oral midodrine treatment accelerates the liberation of intensive care unit patients from intravenous vasopressor infusions. J Crit Care. 2013 Oct;28(5):756-62. doi: 10.1016/j.jcrc.2013.05.021. Epub 2013 Jul 8. PMID: 23845791.
9. Poveromo LB, Michalets EL, Sutherland SE. Midodrine for the weaning of vasopressor infusions. J Clin Pharm Ther. 2016 Jun;41(3):260-5. doi: 10.1111/jcpt.12375. Epub 2016 Mar 4. PMID: 26945564.
10. Santer P, Anstey MH, Patrocínio MD, Wibrow B, Teja B, Shay D, Shaefi S, Parsons CS, Houle TT, Eikermann M; MIDAS Study Group. Effect of midodrine versus placebo on time to vasopressor discontinuation in patients with persistent hypotension in the intensive care unit (MIDAS): an international randomised clinical trial. Intensive Care Med. 2020 Oct;46(10):1884-1893. doi: 10.1007/s00134-020-06216-x. Epub 2020 Sep 3. PMID: 32885276; PMCID: PMC8273663.
11. Costa-Pinto R, Yong ZT, Yanase F, Young C, Brown A, Udy A, Young PJ, Eastwood G, Bellomo R. A pilot, feasibility, randomised controlled trial of midodrine as adjunctive vasopressor for low-dose vasopressor-dependent hypotension in intensive care patients: The MAVERIC study. J Crit Care. 2022 Feb;67:166-171. doi: 10.1016/j.jcrc.2021.11.004. Epub 2021 Nov 18. PMID: 34801917.
12. Prakash S, Garg AX, Heidenheim AP, House AA. Midodrine appears to be safe and effective for dialysis-induced hypotension: a systematic review. Nephrol Dial Transplant. 2004 Oct;19(10):2553-8. doi: 10.1093/ndt/gfh420. Epub 2004 Jul 27. PMID: 15280522.
13. Angeli P, Volpin R, Gerunda G, Craighero R, Roner P, Merenda R, Amodio P, Sticca A, Caregaro L, Maffei-Faccioli A, Gatta A. Reversal of type 1 hepatorenal syndrome with the administration of midodrine and octreotide. Hepatology. 1999 Jun;29(6):1690-7. doi: 10.1002/hep.510290629. PMID: 10347109.
14. Kalambokis G, Fotopoulos A, Economou M, Pappas K, Tsianos EV. Effects of a 7-day treatment with midodrine in non-azotemic cirrhotic patients with and without ascites. J Hepatol. 2007 Feb;46(2):213-21. doi: 10.1016/j.jhep.2006.09.012. Epub 2006 Nov 10. PMID: 17156883.
15. Santer P, Eikermann M. High-dose midodrine is not effective for treatment of persistent hypotension in the intensive care unit. Intensive Care Med. 2021 Feb;47(2):252-253. doi: 10.1007/s00134-020-06333-7. Epub 2021 Jan 8. PMID: 33416917.
6. Mazzeffi M, Hammer B, Chen E, Caridi-Scheible M, Ramsay J, Paciullo C. Methylene blue for postcardiopulmonary bypass vasoplegic syndrome: A cohort study. Ann Card Anaesth. 2017 Apr-Jun;20(2):178-181. doi: 10.4103/aca.ACA_237_16. PMID: 28393777; PMCID: PMC5408522.
7. Tremblay JA, Laramée P, Lamarche Y, Denault A, Beaubien-Souligny W, Frenette AJ, Kontar L, Serri K, Charbonney E. Potential risks in using midodrine for persistent hypotension after cardiac surgery: a comparative cohort study. Ann Intensive Care. 2020 Sep 14;10(1):121. doi: 10.1186/s13613-020-00737-w. PMID: 32926256; PMCID: PMC7490305.
8. Rizvi MS, Nei AM, Gajic O, Mara KC, Barreto EF. Continuation of Newly Initiated Midodrine Therapy After Intensive Care and Hospital Discharge: A Single-Center Retrospective Study. Crit Care Med. 2019 Aug;47(8):e648-e653. doi: 10.1097/CCM.0000000000003814. PMID: 31107279.
9. Teja B, Bosch NA, Walkey AJ. How We Escalate Vasopressor and Corticosteroid Therapy in Patients With Septic Shock. Chest. 2023 Mar;163(3):567-574. doi: 10.1016/j.chest.2022.09.019. Epub 2022 Sep 23. PMID: 36162481.
0. Reed BN, Gale SE, Ramani G. Continuation of Newly Initiated Midodrine Therapy: Appropriate in Patients With Heart Failure? Crit Care Med. 2019 Oct;47(10):e845. doi: 10.1097/CCM.0000000000003914. PMID: 31524705.
1. Steinbach K, Weidinger P. Der Einflubb von Midodrin auf die Orthostase [Effect of midodrin on orthostasis]. Wien Klin Wochenschr. 1973 Sep 21;85(38):621-4. German. PMID: 4148067.
2. Schramek G, Wolkerstorfer H. Zur Therapie der konstitutionellen Hypotonie. Erfahrungen mit Midodrin [Therapy of constitutional hypotension. Experiences with midodrin]. Wien Med Wochenschr. 1973 Sep 29;123(39):571-3. German. PMID: 4748156.
3. Mitka M. Trials to address efficacy of midodrine 18 years after it gains FDA approval. JAMA. 2012 Mar 21;307(11):1124, 1127. doi: 10.1001/jama.2012.291. PMID: 22436941.
4. Angeli P, Volpin R, Gerunda G, Craighero R, Roner P, Merenda R, Amodio P, Sticca A, Caregaro L, Maffei-Faccioli A, Gatta A. Reversal of type 1 hepatorenal syndrome with the administration of midodrine and octreotide. Hepatology. 1999 Jun;29(6):1690-7. doi: 10.1002/hep.510290629. PMID: 10347109.
5. Sharma S, Lardizabal JA, Bhambi B. Oral midodrine is effective for the treatment of hypotension associated with carotid artery stenting. J Cardiovasc Pharmacol Ther. 2008 Jun;13(2):94-7. doi: 10.1177/1074248408317709. PMID: 18495904.

26. Jensen BC, O'Connell TD, Simpson PC. Alpha-1-adrenergic receptors: targets for agonist drugs to treat heart failure. J Mol Cell Cardiol. 2011 Oct;51(4):518-28. doi: 10.1016/j.yjmcc.2010.11.014. Epub 2010 Nov 28. PMID: 21118696; PMCID: PMC3085055.
27. Sharma S, Bhambi B. Successful treatment of hypotension associated with stunned myocardium with oral midodrine therapy. J Cardiovasc Pharmacol Ther. 2005 Mar;10(1):77-9. doi: 10.1177/107424840501000109. PMID: 15821841.

ISOPROTERENOL

1. Panchal AR, Bartos JA, Cabañas JG, Donnino MW, Drennan IR, Hirsch KG, Kudenchuk PJ, Kurz MC, Lavonas EJ, Morley PT, O'Neil BJ, Peberdy MA, Rittenberger JC, Rodriguez AJ, Sawyer KN, Berg KM; Adult Basic and Advanced Life Support Writing Group. Part 3: Adult Basic and Advanced Life Support: 2020 American Heart Association Guidelines for Cardiopulmonary Resuscitation and Emergency Cardiovascular Care. Circulation. 2020 Oct 20;142(16_suppl_2):S366-S468. doi: 10.1161/CIR.0000000000000916. Epub 2020 Oct 21. PMID: 33081529.
2. Gold MI. Treatment of bronchospasm during anesthesia. Anesth Analg. 1975 Nov-Dec;54(6):783-6. PMID: 1239218
3. Herman JJ, Noah ZL, Moody RR. Use of intravenous isoproterenol for status asthmaticus in children. Crit Care Med. 1983 Sep;11(9):716-20. doi: 10.1097/00003246-198309000-00009. PMID: 6884052.
4. Mark AL, Abboud FM, Schmid PG, Heistad DD, Mayer HE. Differences in direct effects of adrenergic stimuli on coronary, cutaneous, and muscular vessels. J Clin Invest. 1972 Feb;51(2):279-87. doi: 10.1172/JCI106812. PMID: 4400290; PMCID: PMC302125.
5. McRaven DR, Mark AL, Abboud FM, Mayer HE. Responses of coronary vessels to adrenergic stimuli. J Clin Invest. 1971 Apr;50(4):773-8. doi: 10.1172/JCI106548. PMID: 4396052; PMCID: PMC291991.
6. Shettigar UR, Hultgren HN, Specter M, Martin R, Davies DH. Primary pulmonary hypertension favorable effect of isoproterenol. N Engl J Med. 1976 Dec 16;295(25):1414-5. doi: 10.1056/NEJM197612162952506. PMID: 980096.
7. Kislitsina ON, Rich JD, Wilcox JE, Pham DT, Churyla A, Vorovich EB, Ghafourian K, Yancy CW. Shock - Classification and Pathophysiological Principles of Therapeutics. Curr Cardiol Rev. 2019;15(2):102-113. doi: 10.2174/1573403X15666181212125024. PMID: 30543176; PMCID: PMC6520577.
8. van Diepen S, Katz JN, Albert NM, Henry TD, Jacobs AK, Kapur NK, Kilic A, Menon V, Ohman EM, Sweitzer NK, Thiele H, Washam JB, Cohen MG; American Heart Association Council on Clinical Cardiology; Council on Cardiovascular and Stroke Nursing; Council on Quality of Care and Outcomes Research; and Mission: Lifeline. Contemporary Management of Cardiogenic Shock: A Scientific Statement From the American Heart Association. Circulation. 2017 Oct 17;136(16):e232-e268. doi: 10.1161/CIR.0000000000000525. Epub 2017 Sep 18. PMID: 28923988.
9. McGAFF CJ, COHEN NK, LEIGHT L. Hemodynamic effects of isoproterenol in complete heart block. AMA Arch Intern Med. 1959 Aug;104(2):242-8. doi: 10.1001/archinte.1959.00270080068008. PMID: 13669778.
10. Morgan DJ. Clinical pharmacokinetics of beta-agonists. Clin Pharmacokinet. 1990 Apr;18(4):270-94. doi: 10.2165/00003088-199018040-00002. PMID: 1969785.
11. SEGAL MS, BEAKEY JF. The use of isuprel for the management of bronchial asthma. Bull New Engl Med Cent. 1947 Apr;9(2):62-7. PMID: 20291309.
12. CHANDLER D, ROSENBAUM J. Severe Adams-Stokes syndrome treated with isuprel and an artificial pacemaker. Am Heart J. 1955 Feb;49(2):295-301. doi: 10.1016/0002-8703(55)90204-0. PMID: 13228364.
13. ECKSTEIN JW, HAMILTON WK. Effects of isoproterenol on peripheral venous tone and transmural right atrial pressure in man. J Clin Invest. 1959 Feb;38(2):342-6. doi: 10.1172/JCI103807. PMID: 13631065; PMCID: PMC293161.
14. Khot UN, Vogan ED, Militello MA. Nitroprusside and Isoproterenol Use after Major Price Increases. N Engl J Med. 2017 Aug 10;377(6):594-595. doi: 10.1056/NEJMc1700244. PMID: 28792879.
15. Puri PS. Modification of experimental myocardial infarct size by cardiac drugs. Am J Cardiol. 1974 Apr;33(4):521-8 doi: 10.1016/0002-9149(74)90612-2. PMID: 4818050.
16. BECKER DJ, NONKIN PM, BENNET LD, KIMBALL SG, STERNBERG MS, WASSERMAN F. Effect of isoproterenol in digitalis cardiotoxicity. Am J Cardiol. 1962 Aug;10:242-7. doi: 10.1016/0002-9149(62)90302-8. PMID: 13866318.
17. Evans L, Rhodes A, Alhazzani W, Antonelli M, Coopersmith CM, French C, Machado FR, Mcintyre L, Ostermann M, Prescott HC, Schorr C, Simpson S, Joost Wiersinga W, Alshamsi F, Angus DC, Arabi Y, Azevedo L, Beale R, Beilman G, Belley-Cote E, Burry L, Cecconi M, Centofanti J, Yataco AC, De Waele J, Dellinger RP, Doi K, Du B, Estenssoro E, Ferrer R, Gomersall C, Hodgson C, Moller MH, Iwashyna T, Jacob S, Kleinpell R, Klompas M, Koh Y, Kumar A, Kwizera A, Lobo S, Masur H, McGloughlin S, Mehta S, Mehta Y, Mer M, Nunnally M, Oczkowski S, Osborn T, Papathanassoglou E, Perner A, Puskarich M, Roberts J, Schweickert W, Seckel M, Sevransky J, Sprung CL, Welte T, Zimmerman J, Levy M. Executive Summary: Surviving Sepsis Campaign: International Guidelines for the Management of Sepsis and Septic Shock 2021. Crit Care Med. 2021 Nov 1;49(11):1974-1982. doi: 10.1097/CCM.0000000000005357. Erratum in: Crit Care Med. 2022 Apr 1;50(4):e413-e414. PMID: 34643578.
18. Leone M, Boyadjiev I, Boulos E, Antonini F, Visintini P, Albanèse J, Martin C. A reappraisal of isoproterenol in goal-directed therapy of septic shock. Shock. 2006 Oct;26(4):353-7. doi: 10.1097/01.shk.0000226345.55657.66. PMID: 16980881.
19. CORCORAN AC, PAGE IH. Renal hemodynamic effects of adrenaline and isuprel; potentiation of effects of both drugs by tetraethyl-ammonium. Proc Soc Exp Biol Med. 1947 Oct;66(1):148-51. doi: 10.3181/00379727-66-16013. PMID: 20270704.
20. Isoproterenol [package insert]. Valeant Pharmaceuticals North America LLC; August 2021.

DOBUTAMINE

1. Scheeren TWL, Bakker J, Kaufmann T, Annane D, Asfar P, Boerma EC, Cecconi M, Chew MS, Cholley B, Cronhjort M, De Backer D, Dubin A, Dünser MW, Duranteau J, Gordon AC, Hajjar LA, Hamzaoui O, Hernandez G, Kanoore Edul V, Koster G, Landoni G, Leone M, Levy B, Martin C, Mebazaa A, Monnet X, Morelli A, Payen D, Pearse RM, Pinsky MR, Radermacher P, Reuter DA, Sakr Y, Sander M, Saugel B, Singer M, Squara P, Vieillard-Baron A, Vignon P, Vincent JL, van der Horst ICC, Vistisen ST, Teboul JL. Current use of inotropes in circulatory shock. Ann Intensive Care. 2021 Jan 29;11(1):21. doi: 10.1186/s13613-021-00806-8. PMID: 33512597; PMCID: PMC7846624.
2. Hollenberg SM. Vasoactive drugs in circulatory shock. Am J Respir Crit Care Med. 2011 Apr 1;183(7):847-55. doi: 10.1164/rccm.201006-0972CI. Epub 2010 Nov 19. PMID: 21097695.
3. Ruffolo RR Jr. The pharmacology of dobutamine. Am J Med Sci. 1987 Oct;294(4):244-8. doi: 10.1097/00000441-198710000-00005. PMID: 3310640.
4. Kislitsina ON, Rich JD, Wilcox JE, Pham DT, Churyla A, Vorovich EB, Ghafourian K, Yancy CW. Shock - Classification and Pathophysiological Principles of Therapeutics. Curr Cardiol Rev. 2019;15(2):102-113. doi: 10.2174/1573403X15666181212125024. PMID: 30543176; PMCID: PMC6520577.
5. Lescroart M, Pequignot B, Janah D, Levy B. The medical treatment of cardiogenic shock. J Intensive Med. 2023 Jan 19;3(2):114-123. doi: 10.1016/j.jointm.2022.12.001. PMID: 37188116; PMCID: PMC10175741.
6. Jentzer JC, Coons JC, Link CB, Schmidhofer M. Pharmacotherapy update on the use of vasopressors and inotropes in the intensive care unit. J Cardiovasc Pharmacol Ther. 2015 May;20(3):249-60. doi: 10.1177/1074248414559838. Epub 2014 Nov 28. PMID: 25432872.
7. van Diepen S, Katz JN, Albert NM, Henry TD, Jacobs AK, Kapur NK, Kilic A, Menon V, Ohman EM, Sweitzer NK, Thiele H, Washam JB, Cohen MG; American Heart Association Council on Clinical Cardiology; Council on Cardiovascular and Stroke Nursing; Council on Quality of Care and Outcomes Research; and Mission: Lifeline. Contemporary Management of Cardiogenic Shock: A Scientific Statement From the American Heart Association. Circulation. 2017 Oct 17;136(16):e232-e268. doi: 10.1161/CIR.0000000000000525. Epub 2017 Sep 18. PMID: 28923988.
8. Shabana A, Dholoo F, Banerjee P. Inotropic Agents and Vasopressors in the Treatment of Cardiogenic Shock. Curr Heart Fail Rep. 2020 Dec;17(6):438-448. doi: 10.1007/s11897-020-00493-9. Epub 2020 Oct 26. PMID: 33103204.
9. Romson JL, Leung JM, Bellows WH, Bronstein M, Keith F, Moores W, Flachsbart K, Richter R, Pastor D, Fisher DM. Effects of dobutamine on hemodynamics and left ventricular performance after cardiopulmonary bypass in cardiac surgical patients. Anesthesiology. 1999 Nov;91(5):1318-28. doi: 10.1097/00000542-199911000-00024. Erratum in: Anesthesiology 2000 Jan;92(1):296. PMID: 10551583.
10. Tamaki Y, Yaku H, Morimoto T, Inuzuka Y, Ozasa N, Yamamoto E, Yoshikawa Y, Miyake M, Kondo H, Tamura T, Kitai T, Iguchi M, Nagao K, Nishikawa R, Kawase Y, Morinaga T, Kawato M, Toyofuku M, Sato Y, Kuwahara K, Nakagawa Y, Kato T, Kimura T; KCHF Study Investigators. Lower In-Hospital Mortality With Beta-Blocker Use at Admission in Patients With Acute Decompensated Heart Failure. J Am Heart Assoc. 2021 Jul 6;10(13):e020012. doi: 10.1161/JAHA.120.020012. Epub 2021 Jun 26. PMID: 34180244; PMCID: PMC8403288.
11. Hospira Pharmaceuticals. Dobutamine (Package Insert). U.S. Food and Drug Administration website. https://www.accessdata.fda.gov/drugsatfda_docs/label/2016/020201s036lbl.pdf. Revised May 2016. Accessed November 2023.
12. Tacon CL, McCaffrey J, Delaney A. Dobutamine for patients with severe heart failure: a systematic review and meta-analysis of randomised controlled trials. Intensive Care Med. 2012 Mar;38(3):359-67. doi: 10.1007/s00134-011-2435-6. Epub 2011 Dec 8. PMID: 22160239.
13. Metra M, Nodari S, D'Aloia A, Muneretto C, Robertson AD, Bristow MR, Dei Cas L. Beta-blocker therapy influences the hemodynamic response to inotropic agents in patients with heart failure: a randomized comparison of dobutamine and enoximone before and after chronic treatment with metoprolol or carvedilol. J Am Coll Cardiol. 2002 Oct 2;40(7):1248-58. doi: 10.1016/s0735-1097(02)02134-4. PMID: 12383572.
14. Lowes BD, Tsvetkova T, Eichhorn EJ, Gilbert EM, Bristow MR. Milrinone versus dobutamine in heart failure subjects treated chronically with carvedilol. Int J Cardiol. 2001 Dec;81(2-3):141-9. doi: 10.1016/s0167-5273(01)00520-4. PMID: 11744130.
15. Overgaard CB, Dzavík V. Inotropes and vasopressors: review of physiology and clinical use in cardiovascular disease. Circulation. 2008 Sep 2;118(10):1047-56. doi: 10.1161/CIRCULATIONAHA.107.728840. PMID: 18765387.
16. Uhlig K, Efremov L, Tongers J, Frantz S, Mikolajczyk R, Sedding D, Schumann J. Inotropic agents and vasodilator strategies for the treatment of cardiogenic shock or low cardiac output syndrome. Cochrane Database Syst Rev. 2020 Nov 5;11(11):CD009669. doi: 10.1002/14651858.CD009669.pub4. PMID: 33152122; PMCID: PMC8094388.
17. Faggiano P, D'Aloia A, Gualeni A, Ambrosino N, Pagani M, Giordano A. Dobutamine-induced changes in pulmonary artery pressure in patients with congestive heart failure and their relation to abnormalities of lung diffusing capacity. Am J Cardiol. 1998 Nov 15;82(10):1296-8, A10. doi: 10.1016/s0002-9149(98)00622-5. PMID: 9832114.
18. Eichhorn EJ, Konstam MA, Weiland DS, Roberts DJ, Martin TT, Stransky NB, Salem DN. Differential effects of milrinone and dobutamine on right ventricular preload, afterload and systolic performance in congestive heart failure secondary to ischemic or idiopathic dilated cardiomyopathy. Am J Cardiol. 1987 Dec 1;60(16):1329-33. doi: 10.1016/0002-9149(87)90616-3. PMID: 3687783.
19. Petersen JW, Felker GM. Inotropes in the management of acute heart failure. Crit Care Med. 2008 Jan;36(1 Suppl):S106-11. doi: 10.1097/01.CCM.0000296273.72952.39. PMID: 18158469.
20. Mager G, Klocke RK, Kux A, Höpp HW, Hilger HH. Phosphodiesterase III inhibition or adrenoreceptor stimulation: milrinone as an alternative to dobutamine in the treatment of severe heart failure. Am Heart J. 1991 Jun;121(6 Pt 2):1974-83. doi: 10.1016/0002-8703(91)90834-5. PMID: 1852090.

21. Prielipp RC, MacGregor DA, Royster RL, Kon ND, Hines MH, Butterworth JF 4th. Dobutamine antagonizes epinephrine's biochemical and cardiotonic effects: results of an in vitro model using human lymphocytes and a clinical study in patients recovering from cardiac surgery. Anesthesiology. 1998 Jul;89(1):49-57. doi: 10.1097/00000542-199807000-00010. PMID: 9667293.
22. Unverferth DA, Blanford M, Kates RE, Leier CV. Tolerance to dobutamine after a 72 hour continuous infusion. Am J Med. 1980 Aug;69(2):262-6. doi: 10.1016/0002-9343(80)90387-3. PMID: 7405947.
23. Evans L, Rhodes A, Alhazzani W, Antonelli M, Coopersmith CM, French C, Machado FR, Mcintyre L, Ostermann M, Prescott HC, Schorr C, Simpson S, Wiersinga WJ, Alshamsi F, Angus DC, Arabi Y, Azevedo L, Beale R, Beilman G, Belley-Cote E, Burry L, Cecconi M, Centofanti J, Coz Yataco A, De Waele J, Dellinger RP, Doi K, Du B, Estenssoro E, Ferrer R, Gomersall C, Hodgson C, Møller MH, Iwashyna T, Jacob S, Kleinpell R, Klompas M, Koh Y, Kumar A, Kwizera A, Lobo S, Masur H, McGloughlin S, Mehta S, Mehta Y, Mer M, Nunnally M, Oczkowski S, Osborn T, Papathanassoglou E, Perner A, Puskarich M, Roberts J, Schweickert W, Seckel M, Sevransky J, Sprung CL, Welte T, Zimmerman J, Levy M. Surviving sepsis campaign: international guidelines for management of sepsis and septic shock 2021. Intensive Care Med. 2021 Nov;47(11):1181-1247. doi: 10.1007/s00134-021-06506-y. Epub 2021 Oct 2. PMID: 34599691; PMCID: PMC8486643.
24. Hasegawa D, Ishisaka Y, Maeda T, Prasitlumkum N, Nishida K, Dugar S, Sato R. Prevalence and Prognosis of Sepsis-Induced Cardiomyopathy: A Systematic Review and Meta-Analysis. J Intensive Care Med. 2023 Jun 4:8850666231180526. doi: 10.1177/08850666231180526. Epub ahead of print. PMID: 37272081.
25. Upadhrasta S, Museedi A, Thannoun T, Chaanine AH, Le Jemtel TH. Early Mechanical Circulatory Support for Cardiogenic Shock. Cardiol Rev. 2023 Jul-Aug 01;31(4):215-218. doi: 10.1097/CRD.0000000000000485. Epub 2022 Oct 25. PMID: 36730923; PMCID: PMC10278569.
26. Annane D, Vignon P, Renault A, Bollaert PE, Charpentier C, Martin C, Troché G, Ricard JD, Nitenberg G, Papazian L, Azoulay E, Bellissant E; CATS Study Group. Norepinephrine plus dobutamine versus epinephrine alone for management of septic shock: a randomised trial. Lancet. 2007 Aug 25;370(9588):676-84. doi: 10.1016/S0140-6736(07)61344-0. Erratum in: Lancet. 2007 Sep 22;370(9592):1034. PMID: 17720019.
27. Farmakis D, Agostoni P, Baholli L, Bautin A, Comin-Colet J, Crespo-Leiro MG, Fedele F, García-Pinilla JM, Giannakoulas G, Grigioni F, Gruchała M, Gustafsson F, Harjola VP, Hasin T, Herpain A, Iliodromitis EK, Karason K, Kivikko M, Liaudet L, Ljubas-Maček J, Marini M, Masip J, Mebazaa A, Nikolaou M, Ostadal P, Põder P, Pollesello P, Polyzogopoulou E, Pölzl G, Tschope C, Varpula M, von Lewinski D, Vrtovec B, Yilmaz MB, Zima E, Parissis J. A pragmatic approach to the use of inotropes for the management of acute and advanced heart failure: An expert panel consensus. Int J Cardiol. 2019 Dec 15;297:83-90. doi: 10.1016/j.ijcard.2019.09.005. Epub 2019 Sep 6. PMID: 31615650.
28. Sarma D, Jentzer J. Cardiogenic Shock: Pathogenesis, Classification, and Management. Critical Care Clinics. Published:July 05, 2023DOI:https://doi.org/10.1016/j.ccc.2023.05.001
29. Levy B, Buzon J, Kimmoun A. Inotropes and vasopressors use in cardiogenic shock: when, which and how much? Curr Opin Crit Care. 2019 Aug;25(4):384-390. doi: 10.1097/MCC.0000000000000632. PMID: 31166204.

MILRINONE
1. Motwani, S. K., and Saunders, H. (2021). Inotropes. Anaesth. Intensive Care Med. 22 (4), 243–248. doi:10.1016/j.mpaic.2021.02.011
2. Bruno RR, Wolff G, Kelm M, Jung C. Pharmacological treatment of cardiogenic shock - A state of the art review. Pharmacol Ther. 2022 Dec;240:108230. doi: 10.1016/j.pharmthera.2022.108230. Epub 2022 Jun 10. PMID: 35697151.
3. Bangash MN, Kong ML, Pearse RM. Use of inotropes and vasopressor agents in critically ill patients. Br J Pharmacol. 2012 Apr;165(7):2015-33. doi: 10.1111/j.1476-5381.2011.01588.x. PMID: 21740415; PMCID: PMC3413841.
4. Bayram M, De Luca L, Massie MB, Gheorghiade M. Reassessment of dobutamine, dopamine, and milrinone in the management of acute heart failure syndromes. Am J Cardiol. 2005 Sep 19;96(6A):47G-58G. doi: 10.1016/j.amjcard.2005.07.021. PMID: 16181823.
5. Kislitsina ON, Rich JD, Wilcox JE, Pham DT, Churyla A, Vorovich EB, Ghafourian K, Yancy CW. Shock - Classification and Pathophysiological Principles of Therapeutics. Curr Cardiol Rev. 2019;15(2):102-113. doi: 10.2174/1573403X15666181212125024. PMID: 30543176; PMCID: PMC6520577.
6. Grose R, Strain J, Greenberg M, LeJemtel TH. Systemic and coronary effects of intravenous milrinone and dobutamine in congestive heart failure. J Am Coll Cardiol. 1986 May;7(5):1107-13. doi: 10.1016/s0735-1097(86)80231-5. PMID: 3958369.
7. Karlsberg RP, DeWood MA, DeMaria AN, Berk MR, Lasher KP. Comparative efficacy of short-term intravenous infusions of milrinone and dobutamine in acute congestive heart failure following acute myocardial infarction. Milrinone-Dobutamine Study Group. Clin Cardiol. 1996 Jan;19(1):21-30. doi: 10.1002/clc.4960190106. PMID: 8903534.
8. Givertz MM, Hare JM, Loh E, Gauthier DF, Colucci WS. Effect of bolus milrinone on hemodynamic variables and pulmonary vascular resistance in patients with severe left ventricular dysfunction: a rapid test for reversibility of pulmonary hypertension. J Am Coll Cardiol. 1996 Dec;28(7):1775-80. doi: 10.1016/S0735-1097(96)00399-3. PMID: 8962566.
9. Botha P, Parry G, Dark JH, Macgowan GA. Acute hemodynamic effects of intravenous sildenafil citrate in congestive heart failure: comparison of phosphodiesterase type-3 and -5 inhibition. J Heart Lung Transplant. 2009 Jul;28(7):676-82. doi: 10.1016/j.healun.2009.04.013. Epub 2009 May 13. PMID: 19560695.

10. Cuffe MS, Califf RM, Adams KF Jr, Benza R, Bourge R, Colucci WS, Massie BM, O'Connor CM, Pina I, Quigg R, Silver MA, Gheorghiade M; Outcomes of a Prospective Trial of Intravenous Milrinone for Exacerbations of Chronic Heart Failure (OPTIME-CHF) Investigators. Short-term intravenous milrinone for acute exacerbation of chronic heart failure: a randomized controlled trial. JAMA. 2002 Mar 27;287(12):1541-7. doi: 10.1001/jama.287.12.1541. PMID: 11911756.

11. Triposkiadis F, Karayannis G, Giamouzis G, Skoularigis J, Louridas G, Butler J. The sympathetic nervous system in heart failure physiology, pathophysiology, and clinical implications. J Am Coll Cardiol. 2009 Nov 3;54(19):1747-62. doi: 10.1016/j.jacc.2009.05.015. PMID: 19874988.

12. Baruch L, Patacsil P, Hameed A, Pina I, Loh E. Pharmacodynamic effects of milrinone with and without a bolus loading infusion. Am Heart J. 2001 Feb;141(2):266-73. doi: 10.1067/mhj.2001.111404. PMID: 11174341.

13. Petersen JW, Felker GM. Inotropes in the management of acute heart failure. Crit Care Med. 2008 Jan;36(1 Suppl):S106-11. doi: 10.1097/01.CCM.0000296273.72952.39. PMID: 18158469.

14. Sanofi-Synthelabo Inc. Primacor - Milrinone (Package Insert). U.S. Food and Drug Administration website. https://www.accessdata.fda.gov/drugsatfda_docs/label/2007/019436s021s022lbl.pdf. Revised January 2003. Accessed November 2023.

15. Valkovec AM, Kram SJ, Henderson JB, Levy JH. Renal Dysfunction and Arrhythmia Association in Patients Receiving Milrinone After Cardiac Surgery. J Cardiothorac Vasc Anesth. 2023 Mar;37(3):353-359. doi: 10.1053/j.jvca.2022.11.027. Epub 2022 Nov 25. PMID: 36566129.

16. Metra M, Nodari S, D'Aloia A, Muneretto C, Robertson AD, Bristow MR, Dei Cas L. Beta-blocker therapy influences the hemodynamic response to inotropic agents in patients with heart failure: a randomized comparison of dobutamine and enoximone before and after chronic treatment with metoprolol or carvedilol. J Am Coll Cardiol. 2002 Oct 2;40(7):1248-58. doi: 10.1016/s0735-1097(02)02134-4. PMID: 12383572.

17. Boldt J, Kling D, Moosdorf R, Hempelmann G. Enoximone treatment of impaired myocardial function during cardiac surgery: combined effects with epinephrine. J Cardiothorac Anesth. 1990 Aug;4(4):462-8. doi: 10.1016/0888-6296(90)90292-n. PMID: 2151889.

18. Royster RL, Butterworth JF 4th, Prielipp RC, Zaloga GP, Lawless SG, Spray BJ, Kon ND, Wallenhaupt SL, Cordell AR. Combined inotropic effects of amrinone and epinephrine after cardiopulmonary bypass in humans. Anesth Analg. 1993 Oct;77(4):662-72. doi: 10.1213/00000539-199310000-00003. PMID: 8214647.

19. Rossinen J, Harjola VP, Siirila-Waris K, Lassus J, Melin J, Peuhkurinen K, Nieminen MS. The use of more than one inotrope in acute heart failure is associated with increased mortality: a multi-centre observational study. Acute Card Care. 2008;10(4):209-13. doi: 10.1080/17482940802262376. PMID: 18720087.

20. Packer M, Carver JR, Rodeheffer RJ, Ivanhoe RJ, DiBianco R, Zeldis SM, Hendrix GH, Bommer WJ, Elkayam U, Kukin ML, et al. Effect of oral milrinone on mortality in severe chronic heart failure. The PROMISE Study Research Group. N Engl J Med. 1991 Nov 21;325(21):1468-75. doi: 10.1056/NEJM199111213252103. PMID: 1944425.

21. Felker GM, Benza RL, Chandler AB, Leimberger JD, Cuffe MS, Califf RM, Gheorghiade M, O'Connor CM; OPTIME-CHF Investigators. Heart failure etiology and response to milrinone in decompensated heart failure: results from the OPTIME-CHF study. J Am Coll Cardiol. 2003 Mar 19;41(6):997-1003. doi: 10.1016/s0735-1097(02)02968-6. PMID: 12651048.

22. Mager G, Klocke RK, Kux A, Höpp HW, Hilger HH. Phosphodiesterase III inhibition or adrenoreceptor stimulation: milrinone as an alternative to dobutamine in the treatment of severe heart failure. Am Heart J. 1991 Jun;121(6 Pt 2):1974-83. doi: 10.1016/0002-8703(91)90834-5. PMID: 1852090.

MILRINONE VS. DOBUTAMINE

1. Mathew R, Di Santo P, Jung RG, Marbach JA, Hutson J, Simard T, Ramirez FD, Harnett DT, Merdad A, Almufleh A, Weng W, Abdel-Razek O, Fernando SM, Kyeremanteng K, Bernick J, Wells GA, Chan V, Froeschl M, Labinaz M, Le May MR, Russo JJ, Hibbert B. Milrinone as Compared with Dobutamine in the Treatment of Cardiogenic Shock. N Engl J Med. 2021 Aug 5;385(6):516-525. doi: 10.1056/NEJMoa2026845. PMID: 34347952.

2. Jung RG, Di Santo P, Mathew R, Simard T, Parlow S, Weng W, Abdel-Razek O, Malhotra N, Cheung M, Hutson JH, Marbach JA, Motazedian P, Thibert MJ, Fernando SM, Nery PB, Nair GM, Russo JJ, Hibbert B, Ramirez FD. Arrhythmic Events and Mortality in Patients With Cardiogenic Shock on Inotropic Support: Results of the DOREMI Randomized Trial. Can J Cardiol. 2023 Apr;39(4):394-402. doi: 10.1016/j.cjca.2022.09.013. Epub 2022 Sep 20. PMID: 36150583.

3. Lowes BD, Tsvetkova T, Eichhorn EJ, Gilbert EM, Bristow MR. Milrinone versus dobutamine in heart failure subjects treated chronically with carvedilol. Int J Cardiol. 2001 Dec;81(2-3):141-9. doi: 10.1016/s0167-5273(01)00520-4. PMID: 11744130.

4. Metra M, Nodari S, D'Aloia A, Muneretto C, Robertson AD, Bristow MR, Dei Cas L. Beta-blocker therapy influences the hemodynamic response to inotropic agents in patients with heart failure: a randomized comparison of dobutamine and enoximone before and after chronic treatment with metoprolol or carvedilol. J Am Coll Cardiol. 2002 Oct 2;40(7):1248-58. doi: 10.1016/s0735-1097(02)02134-4. PMID: 12383572.

5. Schoonen A, van Klei WA, van Wolfswinkel L, van Loon K. Definitions of low cardiac output syndrome after cardiac surgery and their effect on the incidence of intraoperative LCOS: A literature review and cohort study. Front Cardiovasc Med. 2022 Sep 29;9:926957. doi: 10.3389/fcvm.2022.926957. PMID: 36247457; PMCID: PMC9558721.

6. Atallah G, George M, Lehot JJ, Bastien O, Bejuit R, Durand PG, Estanove S. Arythmies chez les patients en bas débit cardiaque après chirurgie valvulaire. Etude randomisée, aveugle et comparative dobutamine versus énoxinone [Arrhythmia in patients with low cardiac output after valvular surgery. Randomized, double-blind comparative study of dobutamine versus enoximone]. Arch Mal Coeur Vaiss. 1990 Sep;83 Spec No 3:63-8. French. PMID: 2147837.

7. Lançon JP, Caillard B, Volot F, Obadia JF, Bock F. Comparaison de l'enoximone et de la dobutamine dans le traitement du bas débit cardiaque après chirurgie cardiaque [Comparison of enoximone versus tobutamine in the treatment of low cardiac output after cardiac surgery]. Ann Fr Anesth Reanim. 1990;9(3):289-94. French. doi: 10.1016/s0750-7658(05)80189-3. Erratum in: Ann Fr Anesth Reanim 1990;9(5):VIII. PMID: 2142589.
8. Feneck RO, Sherry KM, Withington PS, Oduro-Dominah A; European Milrinone Multicenter Trial Group. Comparison of the hemodynamic effects of milrinone with dobutamine in patients after cardiac surgery. J Cardiothorac Vasc Anesth. 2001 Jun;15(3):306-15. doi: 10.1053/jcan.2001.23274. PMID: 11426360.
9. Uhlig K, Efremov L, Tongers J, Frantz S, Mikolajczyk R, Sedding D, Schumann J. Inotropic agents and vasodilator strategies for the treatment of cardiogenic shock or low cardiac output syndrome. Cochrane Database Syst Rev. 2020 Nov 5;11(11):CD009669. doi: 10.1002/14651858.CD009669.pub4. PMID: 33152122; PMCID: PMC8094388.
10. Eskandr AM, Metwally AA, Abu Elkassem MS, Sadik SA, Elmiligy AE, Mourad M, Hussein L. Dobutamine and Nitroglycerin Versus Milrinone for Perioperative Management of Pulmonary Hypertension in Mitral Valve Surgery. A Randomized Controlled Study. J Cardiothorac Vasc Anesth. 2018 Dec;32(6):2540-2546. doi: 10.1053/j.jvca.2018.04.032. Epub 2018 Apr 18. PMID: 29880427.
11. Lewis TC, Aberle C, Altshuler D, Piper GL, Papadopoulos J. Comparative Effectiveness and Safety Between Milrinone or Dobutamine as Initial Inotrope Therapy in Cardiogenic Shock. J Cardiovasc Pharmacol Ther. 2019 Mar;24(2):130-138. doi: 10.1177/1074248418797357. Epub 2018 Sep 2. PMID: 30175599.
12. Alkadri J, Hu R, Jeffers MS, Ross J, McIsaac DI, McDonald B. Comparison of milrinone with dobutamine in cardiac surgery: a systematic review and meta-analysis. Can J Anaesth. 2023 Jul;70(7):1272-1274. doi: 10.1007/s12630-023-02482-7. Epub 2023 May 9. PMID: 37160823.
13. Aranda JM Jr, Schofield RS, Pauly DF, Cleeton TS, Walker TC, Monroe VS Jr, Leach D, Lopez LM, Hill JA. Comparison of dobutamine versus milrinone therapy in hospitalized patients awaiting cardiac transplantation: a prospective, randomized trial. Am Heart J. 2003 Feb;145(2):324-9. doi: 10.1067/mhj.2003.50. PMID: 12595851.
14. Sami F, Acharya P, Noonan G, Maurides S, Al-Masry AA, Bajwa S, Parimi N, Boda I, Tran C, Goyal A, Mastoris I, Dalia T, Sauer A, Bakel AV, Shah Z. Palliative Inotropes in Advanced Heart Failure: Comparing Outcomes Between Milrinone and Dobutamine. J Card Fail. 2022 Dec;28(12):1683-1691. doi: 10.1016/j.cardfail.2022.08.007. Epub 2022 Sep 17. PMID: 36122816.
15. Mathew R, Visintini SM, Ramirez FD, DiSanto P, Simard T, Labinaz M, Hibbert BM. Efficacy of milrinone and dobutamine in low cardiac output states: Systematic review and meta-analysis. Clin Invest Med. 2019 Jun 23;42(2):E26-32. doi: 10.25011/cim.v42i2.32813. PMID: 31228965.

LEVOSIMENDAN

1. Evans L, Rhodes A, Alhazzani W, Antonelli M, Coopersmith CM, French C, Machado FR, Mcintyre L, Ostermann M, Prescott HC, Schorr C, Simpson S, Wiersinga WJ, Alshamsi F, Angus DC, Arabi Y, Azevedo L, Beale R, Beilman G, Belley-Cote E, Burry L, Cecconi M, Centofanti J, Coz Yataco A, De Waele J, Dellinger RP, Doi K, Du B, Estenssoro E, Ferrer R, Gomersall C, Hodgson C, Møller MH, Iwashyna T, Jacob S, Kleinpell R, Klompas M, Koh Y, Kumar A, Kwizera A, Lobo S, Masur H, McGloughlin S, Mehta S, Mehta Y, Mer M, Nunnally M, Oczkowski S, Osborn T, Papathanassoglou E, Perner A, Puskarich M, Roberts J, Schweickert W, Seckel M, Sevransky J, Sprung CL, Welte T, Zimmerman J, Levy M. Surviving sepsis campaign: international guidelines for management of sepsis and septic shock 2021. Intensive Care Med. 2021 Nov;47(11):1181-1247. doi: 10.1007/s00134-021-06506-y. Epub 2021 Oct 2. PMID: 34599691; PMCID: PMC8486643.
2. Welker CC, Mielke JAR, Ramakrishna H. Levosimendan and Low Cardiac Output After Cardiac Surgery: Analysis of Trial Data. J Cardiothorac Vasc Anesth. 2023 Jul;37(7):1294-1297. doi: 10.1053/j.jvca.2023.03.011. Epub 2023 Mar 13. PMID: 37028989.
3. Kislitsina ON, Rich JD, Wilcox JE, Pham DT, Churyla A, Vorovich EB, Ghafourian K, Yancy CW. Shock - Classification and Pathophysiological Principles of Therapeutics. Curr Cardiol Rev. 2019;15(2):102-113. doi: 10.2174/1573403X15666181212125024. PMID: 30543176; PMCID: PMC6520577.
4. Sun T, Zhang N, Cui N, Wang SH, Ding DX, Li N, Chen N, Yu ZB. Efficacy of Levosimendan in the Treatment of Patients With Severe Septic Cardiomyopathy. J Cardiothorac Vasc Anesth. 2023 Mar;37(3):344-349. doi: 10.1053/j.jvca.2022.10.032. Epub 2022 Nov 6. PMID: 36473763.
5. Gordon AC, Perkins GD, Singer M, McAuley DF, Orme RM, Santhakumaran S, Mason AJ, Cross M, Al-Beidh F, Best-Lane J, Brealey D, Nutt CL, McNamee JJ, Reschreiter H, Breen A, Liu KD, Ashby D. Levosimendan for the Prevention of Acute Organ Dysfunction in Sepsis. N Engl J Med. 2016 Oct 27;375(17):1638-1648. doi: 10.1056/NEJMoa1609409. Epub 2016 Oct 5. PMID: 27705084.
6. Mehta RH, Leimberger JD, van Diepen S, Meza J, Wang A, Jankowich R, Harrison RW, Hay D, Fremes S, Duncan A, Soltesz EG, Luber J, Park S, Argenziano M, Murphy E, Marcel R, Kalavrouziotis D, Nagpal D, Bozinovski J, Toller W, Heringlake M, Goodman SG, Levy JH, Harrington RA, Anstrom KJ, Alexander JH; LEVO-CTS Investigators. Levosimendan in Patients with Left Ventricular Dysfunction Undergoing Cardiac Surgery. N Engl J Med. 2017 May 25;376(21):2032-2042. doi: 10.1056/NEJMoa1616218. Epub 2017 Mar 19. PMID: 28316276.
7. Cholley B, Caruba T, Grosjean S, Amour J, Ouattara A, Villacorta J, Miguet B, Guinet P, Lévy F, Squara P, Aït Hamou N, Carillion A, Boyer J, Boughenou MF, Rosier S, Robin E, Radutoiu M, Durand M, Guidon C, Desebbe O, Charles-Nelson A, Menasché P, Rozec B, Girard C, Fellahi JL, Pirracchio R, Chatellier G; -. Effect of Levosimendan on Low Cardiac Output Syndrome in Patients With Low Ejection Fraction Undergoing Coronary Artery Bypass Grafting With Cardiopulmonary Bypass: The LICORN Randomized Clinical Trial. JAMA. 2017 Aug 8;318(6):548-556. doi: 10.1001/jama.2017.9973. PMID: 28787507; PMCID: PMC5817482.
8. Landoni G, Lomivorotov VV, Alvaro G, Lobreglio R, Pisano A, Guarracino F, Calabrò MG, Grigoryev EV, Likhvantsev VV, Salgado-Filho MF, Bianchi A, Pasyuga VV, Baiocchi M, Pappalardo F, Monaco F, Boboshko VA, Abubakirov MN,

Amantea B, Lembo R, Brazzi L, Verniero L, Bertini P, Scandroglio AM, Bove T, Belletti A, Michienzi MG, Shukevich DL, Zabelina TS, Bellomo R, Zangrillo A; CHEETAH Study Group. Levosimendan for Hemodynamic Support after Cardiac Surgery. N Engl J Med. 2017 May 25;376(21):2021-2031. doi: 10.1056/NEJMoa1616325. Epub 2017 Mar 21. PMID: 28320259.

9. Tholén M, Ricksten SE, Lannemyr L. Effects of levosimendan on renal blood flow and glomerular filtration in patients with acute kidney injury after cardiac surgery: a double blind, randomized placebo-controlled study. Crit Care. 2021 Jun 12;25(1):207. doi: 10.1186/s13054-021-03628-z. PMID: 34118980; PMCID: PMC8199833.

10. Abdel Hamid HA, El-Tohamy SA. Comparison between milrinone and levosimendan infusion in patients with peripartum cardiomyopathy. Ain-Shams J Anaesthesiol [serial online] 2014 [cited 2023 Oct 13];7:114-20. Available from: http://www.asja.eg.net/text.asp?2014/7/2/114/133308

11. Orion Pharmaceuticals. Simdax: Levosimendan (Package Insert). https://www.hpra.ie/img/uploaded/swedocuments/f255c6f4-40a8-4c0f-b034-e20069403900.pdf. Revised February 2022. Accessed November 2023.

12. Chan CC, Lee KT, Ho WJ, Chan YH, Chu PH. Levosimendan use in patients with acute heart failure and reduced ejection fraction with or without severe renal dysfunction in critical cardiac care units: a multi-institution database study. Ann Intensive Care. 2021 Feb 8;11(1):27. doi: 10.1186/s13613-021-00810-y. PMID: 33555483; PMCID: PMC7869075.

13. Hospira Pharmaceuticals. Dobutamine (Package Insert). U.S. Food and Drug Administration website. https://www.accessdata.fda.gov/drugsatfda_docs/label/2016/020201s036lbl.pdf. Revised May 2016. Accessed November 2023.

14. Uhlig K, Efremov L, Tongers J, Frantz S, Mikolajczyk R, Sedding D, Schumann J. Inotropic agents and vasodilator strategies for the treatment of cardiogenic shock or low cardiac output syndrome. Cochrane Database Syst Rev. 2020 Nov 5;11(11):CD009669. doi: 10.1002/14651858.CD009669.pub4. PMID: 33152122; PMCID: PMC8094388.

15. Fuhrmann JT, Schmeisser A, Schulze MR, Wunderlich C, Schoen SP, Rauwolf T, Weinbrenner C, Strasser RH. Levosimendan is superior to enoximone in refractory cardiogenic shock complicating acute myocardial infarction. Crit Care Med. 2008 Aug;36(8):2257-66. doi: 10.1097/CCM.0b013e3181809846. Erratum in: Crit Care Med. 2008 Oct;36(10):2966. PMID: 18664782.

16. Bhattacharjee S, Soni KD, Maitra S, Baidya DK. Levosimendan does not provide mortality benefit over dobutamine in adult patients with septic shock: A meta-analysis of randomized controlled trials. J Clin Anesth. 2017 Jun;39:67-72. doi: 10.1016/j.jclinane.2017.03.011. Epub 2017 Mar 30. PMID: 28494911.

17. Radosevich M, Couture EJ, Nabzdyk C. Levosimendan And Septic Cardiomyopathy: A Key That May Have Found Its Lock? J Cardiothorac Vasc Anesth. 2023 Mar;37(3):350-352. doi: 10.1053/j.jvca.2022.12.012. Epub 2022 Dec 19. PMID: 36609077.

18. Cholley B, Levy B, Fellahi JL, Longrois D, Amour J, Ouattara A, Mebazaa A. Levosimendan in the light of the results of the recent randomized controlled trials: an expert opinion paper. Crit Care. 2019 Nov 29;23(1):385. doi: 10.1186/s13054-019-2674-4. PMID: 31783891; PMCID: PMC6883606.

19. Cholley B, Bojan M, Guillon B, Besnier E, Mattei M, Levy B, Ouattara A, Tafer N, Delmas C, Tonon D, Rozec B, Fellahi JL, Lim P, Labaste F, Roubille F, Caruba T, Mauriat P; ARCOTHOVA study group. Overview of the current use of levosimendan in France: a prospective observational cohort study. Ann Intensive Care. 2023 Aug 8;13(1):69. doi: 10.1186/s13613-023-01164-3. Erratum in: Ann Intensive Care. 2023 Sep 29;13(1):94. PMID: 37552372; PMCID: PMC10409690.

METHYLENE BLUE

1. Weingartner R, Oliveira E, Oliveira ES, Sant'Anna UL, Oliveira RP, Azambuja LA, Friedman G. Blockade of the action of nitric oxide in human septic shock increases systemic vascular resistance and has detrimental effects on pulmonary function after a short infusion of methylene blue. Braz J Med Biol Res. 1999 Dec;32(12):1505-13. doi: 10.1590/s0100-879x1999001200009. PMID: 10585632.

2. Diaz Soto JC, Nabzdyk CGS. Running on (Too Many) Fumes? Gaseous Mediators in Septic Shock: A Possible Role for High-Dose Vitamin B12. Chest. 2023 Feb;163(2):262-263. doi: 10.1016/j.chest.2022.10.012. PMID: 36759109.

3. Muhammad R, Dharmadjati BB, Mulia EPB, Rachmi DA. Vasoplegia: Mechanism and Management Following Cardiopulmonary Bypass. Eurasian J Med. 2022 Feb;54(1):92-99. doi: 10.5152/eurasianjmed.2022.20394. PMID: 35307639; PMCID: PMC9634875.

4. Ozal E, Kuralay E, Yildirim V, Kilic S, Bolcal C, Kücükarslan N, Günay C, Demirkilic U, Tatar H. Preoperative methylene blue administration in patients at high risk for vasoplegic syndrome during cardiac surgery. Ann Thorac Surg. 2005 May;79(5):1615-9. doi: 10.1016/j.athoracsur.2004.10.038. PMID: 15854942.

5. Ibarra-Estrada M, Kattan E, Aguilera-González P, Sandoval-Plascencia L, Rico-Jauregui U, Gómez-Partida CA, Ortiz-Macías IX, López-Pulgarín JA, Chávez-Peña Q, Mijangos-Méndez JC, Aguirre-Avalos G, Hernández G. Early adjunctive methylene blue in patients with septic shock: a randomized controlled trial. Crit Care. 2023 Mar 13;27(1):110. doi: 10.1186/s13054-023-04397-7. PMID: 36915146; PMCID: PMC10010212.

6. Schumacher LD, Blumer V, Chaparro SV. Methylene blue-induced serotonin syndrome after left ventricular assist device implantation: A case report and literature review. J Thorac Cardiovasc Surg. 2017 Sep;154(3):e39-e43. doi: 10.1016/j.jtcvs.2017.05.053. Epub 2017 May 24. PMID: 28655448.

7. Katzianer D, Chism K, Qureshi AM, Watson R, Massey HT, Boyle AJ, Reeves G, Danelich I. Serotonin syndrome following left ventricular assist device implantation: A report and institution-specific strategy for prevention. J Cardiol Cases. 2019 Sep 17;20(6):218-220. doi: 10.1016/j.jccase.2019.09.004. PMID: 31762837; PMCID: PMC6859538.

8. Basta MN. Postoperative Serotonin Syndrome Following Methylene Blue Administration for Vasoplegia After Cardiac Surgery: A Case Report and Review of the Literature. Semin Cardiothorac Vasc Anesth. 2021 Mar;25(1):51-56. doi: 10.1177/1089253220960255. Epub 2020 Sep 21. PMID: 32951524.
9. Cruise C, MacKinnon J, Tough J, Houston P. Comparison of meperidine and pancuronium for the treatment of shivering after cardiac surgery. Can J Anaesth. 1992 Jul;39(6):563-8. doi: 10.1007/BF03008319. PMID: 1643679.
10. Wolvetang T, Janse R, Ter Horst M. Serotonin Syndrome After Methylene Blue Administration During Cardiac Surgery: A Case Report and Review. J Cardiothorac Vasc Anesth. 2016 Aug;30(4):1042-5. doi: 10.1053/j.jvca.2015.11.019. Epub 2015 Dec 1. PMID: 27130452.
11. Katzianer D, Chism K, Qureshi AM, Watson R, Massey HT, Boyle AJ, Reeves G, Danelich I. Serotonin syndrome following left ventricular assist device implantation: A report and institution-specific strategy for prevention. J Cardiol Cases. 2019 Sep 17;20(6):218-220. doi: 10.1016/j.jccase.2019.09.004. PMID: 31762837; PMCID: PMC6859538.
12. Pruna A, Bonaccorso A, Belletti A, Turi S, Di Prima AL, D'amico F, Zangrillo A, Kotani Y, Landoni G. Methylene Blue Reduces Mortality in Critically Ill and Perioperative Patients: A Meta-Analysis of Randomized Trials. J Cardiothorac Vasc Anesth. 2023 Oct 1:S1053-0770(23)00802-9. doi: 10.1053/j.jvca.2023.09.037. Epub ahead of print. PMID: 37880041.
13. Kram SJ, Kram BL, Cook JC, Ohman KL, Ghadimi K. Hydroxocobalamin or Methylene Blue for Vasoplegic Syndrome in Adult Cardiothoracic Surgery. J Cardiothorac Vasc Anesth. 2022 Feb;36(2):469-476. doi: 10.1053/j.jvca.2021.05.042. Epub 2021 May 27. PMID: 34176677.
14. Brokmeier HM, Seelhammer TG, Nei SD, Gerberi DJ, Mara KC, Wittwer ED, Wieruszewski PM. Hydroxocobalamin for Vasodilatory Hypotension in Shock: A Systematic Review With Meta-Analysis for Comparison to Methylene Blue. J Cardiothorac Vasc Anesth. 2023 Sep;37(9):1757-1772. doi: 10.1053/j.jvca.2023.04.006. Epub 2023 Apr 7. PMID: 37147207.
15. Klijian A, Khanna AK, Reddy VS, Friedman B, Ortoleva J, Evans AS, Panwar R, Kroll S, Greenfeld CR, Chatterjee S. Treatment With Angiotensin II Is Associated With Rapid Blood Pressure Response and Vasopressor Sparing in Patients With Vasoplegia After Cardiac Surgery: A Post-Hoc Analysis of Angiotensin II for the Treatment of High-Output Shock (ATHOS-3) Study. J Cardiothorac Vasc Anesth. 2021 Jan;35(1):51-58. doi: 10.1053/j.jvca.2020.08.001. Epub 2020 Aug 7. PMID: 32868152.
16. Robinson DN, McFadzean WA. Pulse oximetry and methylene blue. Anaesthesia. 1990 Oct;45(10):884-5. doi: 10.1111/j.1365-2044.1990.tb14584.x. PMID: 2240510.
17. Eisenkraft JB. Methylene blue and pulse oximetry readings: spruiouser and spuriouser. Anesthesiology. 1988 Jan;68(1):171-2. doi: 10.1097/00000542-198801000-00041. PMID: 3337381.
18. Gachot B, Bedos JP, Veber B, Wolff M, Regnier B. Short-term effects of methylene blue on hemodynamics and gas exchange in humans with septic shock. Intensive Care Med. 1995 Dec;21(12):1027-31. doi: 10.1007/BF01700666. PMID: 8750129.
19. McCartney SL, Duce L, Ghadimi K. Intraoperative vasoplegia: methylene blue to the rescue! Curr Opin Anaesthesiol. 2018 Feb;31(1):43-49. doi: 10.1097/ACO.0000000000000548. PMID: 29176374.
20. Jang DH, Nelson LS, Hoffman RS. Methylene blue for distributive shock: a potential new use of an old antidote. J Med Toxicol. 2013 Sep;9(3):242-9. doi: 10.1007/s13181-013-0298-7. PMID: 23580172; PMCID: PMC3770994.
21. Arevalo VN, Bullerwell ML. Methylene Blue as an Adjunct to Treat Vasoplegia in Patients Undergoing Cardiac Surgery Requiring Cardiopulmonary Bypass: A Literature Review. AANA J. 2018 Dec;86(6):455-463. PMID: 31584419.
22. Puntillo F, Giglio M, Pasqualucci A, Brienza N, Paladini A, Varrassi G. Vasopressor-Sparing Action of Methylene Blue in Severe Sepsis and Shock: A Narrative Review. Adv Ther. 2020 Sep;37(9):3692-3706. doi: 10.1007/s12325-020-01422-x. Epub 2020 Jul 23. PMID: 32705530; PMCID: PMC7444404.
23. Petermichl W, Gruber M, Schoeller I, Allouch K, Graf BM, Zausig YA. The additional use of methylene blue has a decatecholaminisation effect on cardiac vasoplegic syndrome after cardiac surgery. J Cardiothorac Surg. 2021 Jul 28;16(1):205. doi: 10.1186/s13019-021-01579-8. PMID: 34321019; PMCID: PMC8320154.
24. Ortoleva JP, Cobey FC. A Systematic Approach to the Treatment of Vasoplegia Based on Recent Advances in Pharmacotherapy. J Cardiothorac Vasc Anesth. 2019 May;33(5):1310-1314. doi: 10.1053/j.jvca.2018.11.025. Epub 2018 Nov 24. PMID: 30598380.
25. Zhao CC, Zhai YJ, Hu ZJ, Huo Y, Li ZQ, Zhu GJ. Efficacy and safety of methylene blue in patients with vasodilator shock: A systematic review and meta-analysis. Front Med (Lausanne). 2022 Sep 26;9:950596. doi: 10.3389/fmed.2022.950596. PMID: 36237547; PMCID: PMC9552293.
26. Maslow AD, Stearns G, Butala P, Schwartz CS, Gough J, Singh AK. The hemodynamic effects of methylene blue when administered at the onset of cardiopulmonary bypass. Anesth Analg. 2006 Jul;103(1):2-8, table of contents. doi: 10.1213/01.ane.0000221261.25310.fe. Erratum in: Anesth Analg. 2007 Jan;104(1):50. Batula, Parag [corrected to Butala, Parag]. PMID: 16790616.
27. Kirov MY, Evgenov OV, Evgenov NV, Egorina EM, Sovershaev MA, Sveinbjørnsson B, Nedashkovsky EV, Bjertnaes LJ. Infusion of methylene blue in human septic shock: a pilot, randomized, controlled study. Crit Care Med. 2001 Oct;29(10):1860-7. doi: 10.1097/00003246-200110000-00002. PMID: 11588440.
28. Hohlfelder B, Douglas A, Wang L, Wanek M, Bauer SR. Association of Methylene Blue Dosing With Hemodynamic Response for the Treatment of Vasoplegia. J Cardiothorac Vasc Anesth. 2022 Sep;36(9):3543-3550. doi: 10.1053/j.jvca.2022.04.003. Epub 2022 Apr 7. PMID: 35697643.
29. Puntillo F, Giglio M, Pasqualucci A, Brienza N, Paladini A, Varrassi G. Vasopressor-Sparing Action of Methylene Blue in Severe Sepsis and Shock: A Narrative Review. Adv Ther. 2020 Sep;37(9):3692-3706. doi: 10.1007/s12325-020-01422-x. Epub 2020 Jul 23. PMID: 32705530; PMCID: PMC7444404.

30. Mazzeffi M, Hammer B, Chen E, Caridi-Scheible M, Ramsay J, Paciullo C. Methylene blue for postcardiopulmonary bypass vasoplegic syndrome: A cohort study. Ann Card Anaesth. 2017 Apr-Jun;20(2):178-181. doi: 10.4103/aca.ACA_237_16. PMID: 28393777; PMCID: PMC5408522.

31. Busse LW, Barker N, Petersen C. Vasoplegic syndrome following cardiothoracic surgery-review of pathophysiology and update of treatment options. Crit Care. 2020 Feb 4;24(1):36. doi: 10.1186/s13054-020-2743-8. PMID: 32019600; PMCID: PMC7001322.

32. Authors/Task Force members; Windecker S, Kolh P, Alfonso F, Collet JP, Cremer J, Falk V, Filippatos G, Hamm C, Head SJ, Jüni P, Kappetein AP, Kastrati A, Knuuti J, Landmesser U, Laufer G, Neumann FJ, Richter DJ, Schauerte P, Sousa Uva M, Stefanini GG, Taggart DP, Torracca L, Valgimigli M, Wijns W, Witkowski A. 2014 ESC/EACTS Guidelines on myocardial revascularization: The Task Force on Myocardial Revascularization of the European Society of Cardiology (ESC) and the European Association for Cardio-Thoracic Surgery (EACTS)Developed with the special contribution of the European Association of Percutaneous Cardiovascular Interventions (EAPCI). Eur Heart J. 2014 Oct 1;35(37):2541-619. doi: 10.1093/eurheartj/ehu278. Epub 2014 Aug 29. PMID: 25173339.

33. Argenziano M, Chen JM, Choudhri AF, Cullinane S, Garfein E, Weinberg AD, Smith CR Jr, Rose EA, Landry DW, Oz MC. Management of vasodilatory shock after cardiac surgery: identification of predisposing factors and use of a novel pressor agent. J Thorac Cardiovasc Surg. 1998 Dec;116(6):973-80. doi: 10.1016/S0022-5223(98)70049-2. PMID: 9832689.

34. Paciullo CA, McMahon Horner D, Hatton KW, Flynn JD. Methylene blue for the treatment of septic shock. Pharmacotherapy. 2010 Jul;30(7):702-15. doi: 10.1592/phco.30.7.702. PMID: 20575634.

35. Yiu P, Robin J, Pattison CW. Reversal of refractory hypotension with single-dose methylene blue after coronary artery bypass surgery. J Thorac Cardiovasc Surg. 1999 Jul;118(1):195-6. doi: 10.1016/S0022-5223(99)70161-3. PMID: 10384205.

36. Perdhana F, Kloping NA, Witarto AP, Nugraha D, Yogiswara N, Luke K, Kloping YP, Rehatta NM. Methylene blue for vasoplegic syndrome in cardiopulmonary bypass surgery: A systematic review and meta-analysis. Asian Cardiovasc Thorac Ann. 2021 Oct;29(8):717-728. doi: 10.1177/0218492321998523. Epub 2021 Mar 2. PMID: 33653154.

37. Ortoleva J, Roberts RJ, Devine LT, French A, Kawabori M, Chen F, Shelton K, Dalia AA. Methylene Blue for Vasoplegia During Extracorporeal Membrane Oxygenation Support. J Cardiothorac Vasc Anesth. 2021 Sep;35(9):2694-2699. doi: 10.1053/j.jvca.2020.12.042. Epub 2020 Dec 29. PMID: 33455885.

38. Furnish C, Mueller SW, Kiser TH, Dufficy L, Sullivan B, Beyer JT. Hydroxocobalamin Versus Methylene Blue for Vasoplegic Syndrome in Cardiothoracic Surgery: A Retrospective Cohort. J Cardiothorac Vasc Anesth. 2020 Jul;34(7):1763-1770. doi: 10.1053/j.jvca.2020.01.033. Epub 2020 Jan 23. PMID: 32115360.

39. Methylene blue. Lexicomp online. Hudson, OH, Wolters Kluwer Clinical Drug Information, Inc. Accessed August 16, 2023.

40. Hydroxocobalamin. Lexicomp online. Hudson, OH, Wolters Kluwer Clinical Drug Information, Inc. Accessed August 16, 2023.

41. Burnes ML, Boettcher BT, Woehlck HJ, Zundel MT, Iqbal Z, Pagel PS. Hydroxocobalamin as a Rescue Treatment for Refractory Vasoplegic Syndrome After Prolonged Cardiopulmonary Bypass. J Cardiothorac Vasc Anesth. 2017 Jun;31(3):1012-1014. doi: 10.1053/j.jvca.2016.08.019. Epub 2016 Aug 18. PMID: 27838199.

42. Cai Y, Mack A, Ladlie BL, Martin AK. The use of intravenous hydroxocobalamin as a rescue in methylene blue-resistant vasoplegic syndrome in cardiac surgery. Ann Card Anaesth. 2017 Oct-Dec;20(4):462-464. doi: 10.4103/aca.ACA_88_17. PMID: 28994688; PMCID: PMC5661322.

43. Feih JT, Rinka JRG, Zundel MT. Methylene Blue Monotherapy Compared With Combination Therapy With Hydroxocobalamin for the Treatment of Refractory Vasoplegic Syndrome: ARetrospective Cohort Study. J Cardiothorac Vasc Anesth. 2019 May;33(5):1301-1307. doi: 10.1053/j.jvca.2018.11.020. Epub 2018 Nov 16. PMID: 30606508.

44. Kirov MY, Evgenov OV, Evgenov NV, Egorina EM, Sovershaev MA, Sveinbjørnsson B, Nedashkovsky EV, Bjertnaes LJ. Infusion of methylene blue in human septic shock: a pilot, randomized, controlled study. Crit Care Med. 2001 Oct;29(10):1860-7. doi: 10.1097/00003246-200110000-00002. PMID: 11588440.

45. Memis D, Karamanlioglu B, Yuksel M, Gemlik I, Pamukcu Z. The influence of methylene blue infusion on cytokine levels during severe sepsis. Anaesth Intensive Care. 2002 Dec;30(6):755-62. doi: 10.1177/0310057X0203000606. PMID: 12500513.

46. Mouncey PR, Osborn TM, Power GS, Harrison DA, Sadique MZ, Grieve RD, Jahan R, Harvey SE, Bell D, Bion JF, Coats TJ, Singer M, Young JD, Rowan KM; ProMISe Trial Investigators. Trial of early, goal-directed resuscitation for septic shock. N Engl J Med. 2015 Apr 2;372(14):1301-11. doi: 10.1056/NEJMoa1500896. Epub 2015 Mar 17. PMID: 25776532.

47. ProCESS Investigators; Yealy DM, Kellum JA, Huang DT, Barnato AE, Weissfeld LA, Pike F, Terndrup T, Wang HE, Hou PC, LoVecchio F, Filbin MR, Shapiro NI, Angus DC. A randomized trial of protocol-based care for early septic shock. N Engl J Med. 2014 May 1;370(18):1683-93. doi: 10.1056/NEJMoa1401602. Epub 2014 Mar 18. PMID: 24635773; PMCID: PMC4101700.

48. ARISE Investigators; ANZICS Clinical Trials Group; Peake SL, Delaney A, Bailey M, Bellomo R, Cameron PA, Cooper DJ, Higgins AM, Holdgate A, Howe BD, Webb SA, Williams P. Goal-directed resuscitation for patients with early septic shock. N Engl J Med. 2014 Oct 16;371(16):1496-506. doi: 10.1056/NEJMoa1404380. Epub 2014 Oct 1. PMID: 25272316.

49. Teja B, Bosch NA, Walkey AJ. How We Escalate Vasopressor and Corticosteroid Therapy in Patients With Septic Shock. Chest. 2023 Mar;163(3):567-574. doi: 10.1016/j.chest.2022.09.019. Epub 2022 Sep 23. PMID: 36162481.

50. Jozwiak M. Alternatives to norepinephrine in septic shock: Which agents and when? J Intensive Med. 2022 Jun 12;2(4):223-232. doi: 10.1016/j.jointm.2022.05.001. PMID: 36788938; PMCID: PMC9924015.
51. ProvayBlue® (methylene blue) Injection, USP [package insert]. Shirley, NY: American Regent, Inc.; 12/2021.
52. Leyh RG, Kofidis T, Strüber M, Fischer S, Knobloch K, Wachsmann B, Hagl C, Simon AR, Haverich A. Methylene blue: the drug of choice for catecholamine-refractory vasoplegia after cardiopulmonary bypass? J Thorac Cardiovasc Surg. 2003 Jun;125(6):1426-31. doi: 10.1016/s0022-5223(02)73284-4. PMID: 12830064.
53. Hosseinian L, Weiner M, Levin MA, Fischer GW. Methylene Blue: Magic Bullet for Vasoplegia? Anesth Analg. 2016 Jan;122(1):194-201. doi: 10.1213/ANE.0000000000001045. PMID: 26678471.
54. Jorge-Monjas P, Bardají-Carrillo M, Lorenzo-López M, Tamayo E. Time Matters When Adding Corticosteroids to Escalating Vasopressors in Septic Shock. Chest. 2023 Jul;164(1):e19-e20. doi: 10.1016/j.chest.2023.03.048. PMID: 37423702.
55. Valent P, Groner B, Schumacher U, Superti-Furga G, Busslinger M, Kralovics R, Zielinski C, Penninger JM, Kerjaschki D, Stingl G, Smolen JS, Valenta R, Lassmann H, Kovar H, Jäger U, Kornek G, Müller M, Sörgel F. Paul Ehrlich (1854-1915) and His Contributions to the Foundation and Birth of Translational Medicine. J Innate Immun. 2016;8(2):111-20. doi: 10.1159/000443526. Epub 2016 Feb 5. PMID: 26845587; PMCID: PMC6738855.
56. Juffermans NP, Vervloet MG, Daemen-Gubbels CR, Binnekade JM, de Jong M, Groeneveld AB. A dose-finding study of methylene blue to inhibit nitric oxide actions in the hemodynamics of human septic shock. Nitric Oxide. 2010 May 15;22(4):275-80. doi: 10.1016/j.niox.2010.01.006. Epub 2010 Jan 28. PMID: 20109575.

HYDROXOCOBALAMIN
1. CYANOKIT package insert (single 5-g vial), Columbia, MD: Meridian Medical Technologies, Inc.; 2017
2. Roderique JD, VanDyck K, Holman B, Tang D, Chui B, Spiess BD. The use of high-dose hydroxocobalamin for vasoplegic syndrome. Ann Thorac Surg. 2014 May;97(5):1785-6. doi: 10.1016/j.athoracsur.2013.08.050. PMID: 24792267.
3. Lin Y, Vu TQ. Use of High-Dose Hydroxocobalamin for Septic Shock: A Case Report. A A Pract. 2019 May 1;12(9):332-335. doi: 10.1213/XAA.0000000000000928. PMID: 30431443.
4. Ortoleva JP, Cobey FC. A Systematic Approach to the Treatment of Vasoplegia Based on Recent Advances in Pharmacotherapy. J Cardiothorac Vasc Anesth. 2019 May;33(5):1310-1314. doi: 10.1053/j.jvca.2018.11.025. Epub 2018 Nov 24. PMID: 30598380.
5. Patel JJ, Willoughby R, Peterson J, Carver T, Zelten J, Markiewicz A, Spiegelhoff K, Hipp LA, Canales B, Szabo A, Heyland DK, Stoppe C, Zielonka J, Freed JK. High-Dose IV Hydroxocobalamin (Vitamin B12) in Septic Shock: A Double-Blind, Allocation-Concealed, Placebo-Controlled Single-Center Pilot Randomized Controlled Trial (The Intravenous Hydroxocobalamin in Septic Shock Trial). Chest. 2023 Feb;163(2):303-312. doi: 10.1016/j.chest.2022.09.021. Epub 2022 Sep 26. PMID: 36174744.
6. Burnes ML, Boettcher BT, Woehlck HJ, Zundel MT, Iqbal Z, Pagel PS. Hydroxocobalamin as a Rescue Treatment for Refractory Vasoplegic Syndrome After Prolonged Cardiopulmonary Bypass. J Cardiothorac Vasc Anesth. 2017 Jun;31(3):1012-1014. doi: 10.1053/j.jvca.2016.08.019. Epub 2016 Aug 18. PMID: 27838199.
7. Weinberg JB, Chen Y, Jiang N, Beasley BE, Salerno JC, Ghosh DK. Inhibition of nitric oxide synthase by cobalamins and cobinamides. Free Radic Biol Med. 2009 Jun 15;46(12):1626-32. doi: 10.1016/j.freeradbiomed.2009.03.017. Epub 2009 Mar 27. Erratum in: Free Radic Biol Med. 2011 Oct 1;51(7):1471. PMID: 19328848; PMCID: PMC2745708.
8. Roderique JD, VanDyck K, Holman B, Tang D, Chui B, Spiess BD. The use of high-dose hydroxocobalamin for vasoplegic syndrome. Ann Thorac Surg. 2014 May;97(5):1785-6. doi: 10.1016/j.athoracsur.2013.08.050. PMID: 24792267.
9. Diaz Soto JC, Nabzdyk CGS. Running on (Too Many) Fumes? Gaseous Mediators in Septic Shock: A Possible Role for High-Dose Vitamin B12. Chest. 2023 Feb;163(2):262-263. doi: 10.1016/j.chest.2022.10.012. PMID: 36759109.
10. Shapeton AD, Mahmood F, Ortoleva JP. Hydroxocobalamin for the Treatment of Vasoplegia: A Review of Current Literature and Considerations for Use. J Cardiothorac Vasc Anesth. 2019 Apr;33(4):894-901. doi: 10.1053/j.jvca.2018.08.017. Epub 2018 Aug 11. PMID: 30217583.
11. Busse LW, Barker N, Petersen C. Vasoplegic syndrome following cardiothoracic surgery-review of pathophysiology and update of treatment options. Crit Care. 2020 Feb 4;24(1):36. doi: 10.1186/s13054-020-2743-8. PMID: 32019600; PMCID: PMC7001322.
12. Ortoleva J, Shapeton AD. Seeing Red: Hydroxocobalamin and Result Interference. J Cardiothorac Vasc Anesth. 2023 Aug;37(8):1339-1342. doi: 10.1053/j.jvca.2023.03.017. Epub 2023 Mar 17. PMID: 37120323.
13. Shah PR, Reynolds PS, Pal N, Tang D, McCarthy H, Spiess BD. Hydroxocobalamin for the treatment of cardiac surgery-associated vasoplegia: a case series. Can J Anaesth. 2018 May;65(5):560-568. English. doi: 10.1007/s12630-017-1029-3. Epub 2017 Dec 5. PMID: 29209927.
14. Brokmeier HM, Seelhammer TG, Nei SD, Gerberi DJ, Mara KC, Wittwer ED, Wieruszewski PM. Hydroxocobalamin for Vasodilatory Hypotension in Shock: A Systematic Review With Meta-Analysis for Comparison to Methylene Blue. J Cardiothorac Vasc Anesth. 2023 Sep;37(9):1757-1772. doi: 10.1053/j.jvca.2023.04.006. Epub 2023 Apr 7. PMID: 37147207.
15. Vollmer N, Wieruszewski PM, Martin N, Seelhammer T, Wittwer E, Nabzdyk C, Mara K, Nei SD. Predicting the Response of Hydroxocobalamin in Postoperative Vasoplegia in Recipients of Cardiopulmonary Bypass. J Cardiothorac Vasc Anesth. 2022 Aug;36(8 Pt B):2908-2916. doi: 10.1053/j.jvca.2022.01.021. Epub 2022 Jan 20. PMID: 35181236.

16. Ritter LA, Maldarelli M, McCurdy MT, Yamane DP, Davison D, Parrino C, Yim DN, Lee M, Mazzeffi MA, Chow JH. Effects of a single bolus of hydroxocobalamin on hemodynamics in vasodilatory shock. J Crit Care. 2022 Feb;67:66-71. doi: 10.1016/j.jcrc.2021.09.024. Epub 2021 Oct 21. PMID: 34689063.
17. Sacco AJ, Cunningham CA, Kosiorek HE, Sen A. Hydroxocobalamin in Refractory Septic Shock: A Retrospective Case Series. Crit Care Explor. 2021 Apr 26;3(4):e0408. doi: 10.1097/CCE.0000000000000408. PMID: 33912838; PMCID: PMC8078293.
18. Kumar N, Rahman GR, Falkson S, Lu SY, Dalia A. Hydroxocobalamin in Refractory Vasodilatory Shock: More Questions than Answers. J Cardiothorac Vasc Anesth. 2023 Sep;37(9):1773-1775. doi: 10.1053/j.jvca.2023.05.001. Epub 2023 May 6. PMID: 37225547.
19. Legrand M, Michel T, Daudon M, Benyamina M, Ferry A, Soussi S, Maurel V, Chaussard M, Chaouat M, Mimoun M, Verine J, Mallet V, Mebazaa A; PRONOBURN Study Group. Risk of oxalate nephropathy with the use of cyanide antidote hydroxocobalamin in critically ill burn patients. Intensive Care Med. 2016 Jun;42(6):1080-1. doi: 10.1007/s00134-016-4252-4. Epub 2016 Feb 18. PMID: 26891675.

METHYLENE BLUE VS. HYDROXOCOBALAMIN
1. Furnish C, Mueller SW, Kiser TH, Dufficy L, Sullivan B, Beyer JT. Hydroxocobalamin Versus Methylene Blue for Vasoplegic Syndrome in Cardiothoracic Surgery: A Retrospective Cohort. J Cardiothorac Vasc Anesth. 2020 Jul;34(7):1763-1770. doi: 10.1053/j.jvca.2020.01.033. Epub 2020 Jan 23. PMID: 32115360.
2. Kram SJ, Kram BL, Cook JC, Ohman KL, Ghadimi K. Hydroxocobalamin or Methylene Blue for Vasoplegic Syndrome in Adult Cardiothoracic Surgery. J Cardiothorac Vasc Anesth. 2022 Feb;36(2):469-476. doi: 10.1053/j.jvca.2021.05.042. Epub 2021 May 27. PMID: 34176677.
3. Brokmeier HM, Seelhammer TG, Nei SD, Gerberi DJ, Mara KC, Wittwer ED, Wieruszewski PM. Hydroxocobalamin for Vasodilatory Hypotension in Shock: A Systematic Review With Meta-Analysis for Comparison to Methylene Blue. J Cardiothorac Vasc Anesth. 2023 Sep;37(9):1757-1772. doi: 10.1053/j.jvca.2023.04.006. Epub 2023 Apr 7. PMID: 37147207.
4. Hiruy A, Ciapala S, Donaldson C, Wang L, Hohlfelder B. Hydroxocobalamin Versus Methylene Blue for the Treatment of Vasoplegic Shock Associated With Cardiopulmonary Bypass. J Cardiothorac Vasc Anesth. 2023 Jul 19:S1053-0770(23)00503-7. doi: 10.1053/j.jvca.2023.07.015. Epub ahead of print. PMID: 37586951.
5. Mazzeffi M, Hammer B, Chen E, Caridi-Scheible M, Ramsay J, Paciullo C. Methylene blue for postcardiopulmonary bypass vasoplegic syndrome: A cohort study. Ann Card Anaesth. 2017 Apr-Jun;20(2):178-181. doi: 10.4103/aca.ACA_237_16. PMID: 28393777; PMCID: PMC5408522.
6. Ortoleva J, Roberts RJ, Devine LT, French A, Kawabori M, Chen F, Shelton K, Dalia AA. Methylene Blue for Vasoplegia During Extracorporeal Membrane Oxygenation Support. J Cardiothorac Vasc Anesth. 2021 Sep;35(9):2694-2699. doi: 10.1053/j.jvca.2020.12.042. Epub 2020 Dec 29. PMID: 33455885.
7. Burnes ML, Boettcher BT, Woehlck HJ, Zundel MT, Iqbal Z, Pagel PS. Hydroxocobalamin as a Rescue Treatment for Refractory Vasoplegic Syndrome After Prolonged Cardiopulmonary Bypass. J Cardiothorac Vasc Anesth. 2017 Jun;31(3):1012-1014. doi: 10.1053/j.jvca.2016.08.019. Epub 2016 Aug 18. PMID: 27838199.
8. Cai Y, Mack A, Ladlie BL, Martin AK. The use of intravenous hydroxocobalamin as a rescue in methylene blue-resistant vasoplegic syndrome in cardiac surgery. Ann Card Anaesth. 2017 Oct-Dec;20(4):462-464. doi: 10.4103/aca.ACA_88_17. PMID: 28994688; PMCID: PMC5661322.
9. Feih JT, Rinka JRG, Zundel MT. Methylene Blue Monotherapy Compared With Combination Therapy With Hydroxocobalamin for the Treatment of Refractory Vasoplegic Syndrome: ARetrospective Cohort Study. J Cardiothorac Vasc Anesth. 2019 May;33(5):1301-1307. doi: 10.1053/j.jvca.2018.11.020. Epub 2018 Nov 16. PMID: 30606508.
10. Methylene blue. Lexicomp online. Hudson, OH, Wolters Kluwer Clinical Drug Information, Inc. Accessed August 16, 2023.
11. Hydroxocobalamin. Lexicomp online. Hudson, OH, Wolters Kluwer Clinical Drug Information, Inc. Accessed August 16, 2023.

PERIPHERAL VASOPRESSORS
1. Datar S, Gutierrez E, Schertz A, Vachharajani V. Safety of Phenylephrine Infusion Through Peripheral Intravenous Catheter in the Neurological Intensive Care Unit. J Intensive Care Med. 2018 Oct;33(10):589-592. doi: 10.1177/0885066617712214. Epub 2017 Jun 1. PMID: 28569131.
2. Permpikul C, Tongyoo S, Viarasilpa T, Trainarongsakul T, Chakorn T, Udompanturak S. Early Use of Norepinephrine in Septic Shock Resuscitation (CENSER). A Randomized Trial. Am J Respir Crit Care Med. 2019 May 1;199(9):1097-1105. doi: 10.1164/rccm.201806-1034OC. PMID: 30704260.
3. Ospina-Tascón GA, Hernandez G, Alvarez I, Calderón-Tapia LE, Manzano-Nunez R, Sánchez-Ortiz AI, Quiñones E, Ruiz-Yucuma JE, Aldana JL, Teboul JL, Cavalcanti AB, De Backer D, Bakker J. Effects of very early start of norepinephrine in patients with septic shock: a propensity score-based analysis. Crit Care. 2020 Feb 14;24(1):52. doi: 10.1186/s13054-020-2756-3. PMID: 32059682; PMCID: PMC7023737.
4. McGee DC, Gould MK. Preventing complications of central venous catheterization. N Engl J Med. 2003 Mar 20;348(12):1123-33. doi: 10.1056/NEJMra011883. PMID: 12646670.
5. Parienti JJ, Mongardon N, Mégarbane B, Mira JP, Kalfon P, Gros A, Marqué S, Thuong M, Pottier V, Ramakers M, Savary B, Seguin A, Valette X, Terzi N, Sauneuf B, Cattoir V, Mermel LA, du Cheyron D; 3SITES Study Group. Intravascular Complications of Central Venous Catheterization by Insertion Site. N Engl J Med. 2015 Sep 24;373(13):1220-9. doi: 10.1056/NEJMoa1500964. PMID: 26398070.

6. Owen VS, Rosgen BK, Cherak SJ, Ferland A, Stelfox HT, Fiest KM, Niven DJ. Adverse events associated with administration of vasopressor medications through a peripheral intravenous catheter: a systematic review and meta-analysis. Crit Care. 2021 Apr 16;25(1):146. doi: 10.1186/s13054-021-03553-1. PMID: 33863361; PMCID: PMC8050944.
7. Evans L, Rhodes A, Alhazzani W, Antonelli M, Coopersmith CM, French C, Machado FR, Mcintyre L, Ostermann M, Prescott HC, Schorr C, Simpson S, Wiersinga WJ, Alshamsi F, Angus DC, Arabi Y, Azevedo L, Beale R, Beilman G, Belley-Cote E, Burry L, Cecconi M, Centofanti J, Coz Yataco A, De Waele J, Dellinger RP, Doi K, Du B, Estenssoro E, Ferrer R, Gomersall C, Hodgson C, Møller MH, Iwashyna T, Jacob S, Kleinpell R, Klompas M, Koh Y, Kumar A, Kwizera A, Lobo S, Masur H, McGloughlin S, Mehta S, Mehta Y, Mer M, Nunnally M, Oczkowski S, Osborn T, Papathanassoglou E, Perner A, Puskarich M, Roberts J, Schweickert W, Seckel M, Sevransky J, Sprung CL, Welte T, Zimmerman J, Levy M. Surviving sepsis campaign: international guidelines for management of sepsis and septic shock 2021. Intensive Care Med. 2021 Nov;47(11):1181-1247. doi: 10.1007/s00134-021-06506-y. Epub 2021 Oct 2. PMID: 34599691; PMCID: PMC8486643.
8. Cardenas-Garcia J, Schaub KF, Belchikov YG, Narasimhan M, Koenig SJ, Mayo PH. Safety of peripheral intravenous administration of vasoactive medication. J Hosp Med. 2015 Sep;10(9):581-5. doi: 10.1002/jhm.2394. Epub 2015 May 26. PMID: 26014852.
9. Loubani OM, Green RS. A systematic review of extravasation and local tissue injury from administering vasopressors through peripheral intravenous and central venous catheters. J Crit Care. 2015 Jun;30(3):653.e9-17. doi: 10.1016/j.jcrc.2015.01.014. Epub 2015 Jan 22. PMID: 25669592.
10. Tian DH, Smyth C, Keijzers G, Macdonald SP, Peake S, Udy A, Delaney A. Safety of peripheral administration of vasopressor medications: A systematic review. Emerg Med Australas. 2020 Apr;32(2):220-227. doi: 10.1111/1742-6723.13406. Epub 2019 Nov 7. PMID: 31698544.
11. Lewis T, Merchan C, Altshuler D, Papadopoulos J. Safety of the Peripheral Administration of Vasopressor Agents. J Intensive Care Med. 2019 Jan;34(1):26-33. doi: 10.1177/0885066616686035. Epub 2017 Jan 11. PMID: 28073314.
12. Medlej K, Kazzi AA, El Hajj Chehade A, Saad Eldine M, Chami A, Bachir R, Zebian D, Abou Dagher G. Complications from Administration of Vasopressors Through Peripheral Venous Catheters: An Observational Study. J Emerg Med. 2018 Jan;54(1):47-53. doi: 10.1016/j.jemermed.2017.09.007. Epub 2017 Oct 27. PMID: 29110979.
13. Delgado T, Wolfe B, Davis G, Ansari S. Safety of peripheral administration of phenylephrine in a neurologic intensive care unit: A pilot study. J Crit Care. 2016 Aug;34:107-10. doi: 10.1016/j.jcrc.2016.04.004. Epub 2016 Apr 13. PMID: 27288620.
14. National Institutes of Health (NIH). Common Terminology Criteria for Adverse Events, V5.0. November 2017. Available at: https://ctep.cancer.gov/protocoldevelopment/electronic_applications/docs/ctcae_v5_quick_reference_8.5x11.pdf. Accessed September 5, 2023.
15. EXTRAVASATION. Journal of Infusion Nursing 29(1):p S61-S62, January 2006.
16. Pancaro C, Shah N, Pasma W, Saager L, Cassidy R, van Klei W, Kooij F, Vittali D, Hollmann MW, Kheterpal S, Lirk P. Risk of Major Complications After Perioperative Norepinephrine Infusion Through Peripheral Intravenous Lines in a Multicenter Study. Anesth Analg. 2020 Oct;131(4):1060-1065. doi: 10.1213/ANE.0000000000004445. PMID: 32925324.
17. LEVOPHED package insert, Lake Forest, IL: Hospira, Inc.; 2020.

162

Made in the USA
Las Vegas, NV
27 April 2024